Electrophysiology in Neurotoxicology

Volume II

Editor

Herbert E. Lowndes, Ph.D.
Professor
Department of Pharmacology and Toxicology
Rutgers, The State University of New Jersey
Piscataway, New Jersey

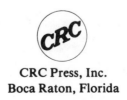

CRC Press, Inc.
Boca Raton, Florida

Library of Congress Cataloging-in-Publication Data

Electrophysiology in neurotoxicology.

Includes bibliographies and index.
1. Neurotoxic agents. 2. Electrophysiology.
I. Lowndes, Herbert E. [DNLM: 1. Electrophysiology.
2. Nervous System—drug effects. 3. Nervous System—
physiology. WL 102 E387]
RC365.E44 1987   615'.78   86-24483
ISBN 0-8493-4693-2 (set)
ISBN 0-8493-4694-0 (v. 1)
ISBN 0-8493-4695-9 (v. 2)

This book represents information obtained from authentic and highly regarded sources. Reprinted material is quoted with permission, and sources are indicated. A wide variety of references are listed. Every reasonable effort has been made to give reliable data and information, but the author and the publisher cannot assume responsibility for the validity of all materials or for the consequences of their use.

Direct all inquiries to CRC Press, Inc., 2000 Corporate Blvd., N.W., Boca Raton, Florida, 33431.

© 1987 by CRC Press, Inc.

International Standard Book Number 0-8493-4693-2 (set)
International Standard Book Number 0-8493-4694-0 (v. 1)
International Standard Book Number 0-8493-4695-9 (v. 2)

Library of Congress Card Number 86-24483
Printed in the United States

PREFACE

The intent in assembling the volume is twofold: first to describe major techniques in sufficient detail as to enable other investigators to implement their use and second, to review the neurotoxicology literature in which the various methodologies have been employed. In some cases, this is accomplished by companion chapters, in others, both aims are achieved in a single chapter. The methodology for clinically used electrophysiological tests has been exhaustively detailed elsewhere and this chapter considers the strengths and limitations of these procedures in human neurotoxicology.

Herbert E. Lowndes

THE EDITOR

Herbert E. Lowndes, Ph.D. is Professor of Pharmacology and Toxicology, College of Pharmacy at Rutgers University, Piscataway, New Jersey. Dr. Lowndes received a B.A. in physics and mathematics (1964) and an M.Sc. in pharmacology (1970) from the University of Saskatchewan, Saskatoon, Canada; a Ph.D. in pharmacology was awarded by Cornell University in 1972. He served as an Assistant Professor through Professor of Pharmacology at New Jersey Medical School from 1973 to 1985.

Dr. Lowndes is a member of 15 professional and/or scientific organizations, an Associate Editor of *Toxicology and Applied Pharmacology,* and a Past-President of the Neurotoxicology Specialty Section, Society of Toxicology. He serves in numerous advisory/consulting roles and is a current recipient of a Jacob Javits Neuroscience Investigator Award from the National Institute of Communicative Disorders and Stroke, National Institutes of Health. His current research interests are in correlative electrophysiological, histochemical, morphological, and immunocytochemical studies of the mechanisms and neurological consequences of toxic chemicals.

CONTRIBUTORS

Rebecca J. Anderson, Ph.D.
Group Leader
Neurological Diseases
Parke-Davis Pharmaceutical Research
  Division
Warner-Lambert Company
Ann Arbor, Michigan

William D. Atchison, Ph.D.
Assistant Professor
Department of Pharmacology and
  Toxicology, and Neuroscience Program
Center for Environmental Toxicology
Michigan State University
East Lansing, Michigan

Thomas Baker, M.S.
Director of Research
Department of Anesthesiology
St. Joseph Hospital and Medical Center
Paterson, New Jersey

George G. Bierkamper, Ph.D.
Associate Professor
Department of Pharmacology
University of Nevada School of Medicine
Reno, Nevada

Robert S. Dyer, Ph.D.
Chief, Neurophysiology Branch
Neurotoxicology Division
U.S. Environmental Protection Agency
Research Triangle Park, North Carolina

Barry D. Goldstein, Ph.D.
Associate Professor
Department of Pharmacology and
  Toxicology
Medical College of Georgia
Augusta, Georgia

Pamela M. Le Quesne, DM. FRCT
Medical School and MRC Toxicology
  Unit
Department of Neurological Studies
The Middlesex Hospital
London WIN8AA, England

Herbert E. Lowndes, Ph.D.
Department of Pharmacology and
  Toxicology
College of Pharmacy
Rutgers, The State University of New
  Jersey
Piscataway, New Jersey

Joseph J. McArdle, Ph.D.
Professor
Department of Pharmacology
UMDNJ-New Jersey Medical School
Newark, New Jersey

Toshio Narahashi, Ph.D.
Alfred Newton Richards Professor and
  Chairman
Department of Pharmacology
Northwestern University Medical School
Chicago, Illinois

TABLE OF CONTENTS

VOLUME I

Chapter 1
Molecular Basis of Signalling in the Nervous System 1
J. J. McArdle

Chapter 2
Effects of Toxic Agents on Neural Membranes 23
T. Narashashi

Chapter 3
Physiology of Synaptic Transmission 45
W. D. Atchison

Chapter 4
Clinically Used Electrophysiological End-points 103
P. M. Le Quesne

Index 117

VOLUME II

Chapter 5
Somatosensory Evoked Potentials 1
R. S. Dyer

Chapter 6
Spinal Cord Reflexes 35
B. D. Goldstein

Chapter 7
Peripheral Nerve Conduction Velocities and Excitability 51
R. J. Anderson

Chapter 8
Sensory Nerve Terminal Function 71
B. D. Goldstein

Chapter 9
Motor Nerve Terminal Responsiveness 87
T. Baker and H. E. Lowndes

Chapter 10
Synaptic Toxicology of Environmental Agents 99
G. Bierkamper

Index 135

Chapter 5

SOMATOSENSORY EVOKED POTENTIALS*

Robert S. Dyer

TABLE OF CONTENTS

I.   Introduction 2

II.   The Phenomenology of SEPs 3
      A.   SEP Peak Nomenclature 4
      B.   Far-Field Potentials 8
      C.   Species Comparisons 10
      D.   Development of the SEP 13
      E.   Gender Differences in SEPs 16

III.   Interpretation of SEPs 17
      A.   Relationship of SEPs to Perception 17
      B.   SEP Changes in Neurological Disorders 18

IV.   Uses of SEPs 21
      A.   Diagnosis and Surgical Monitoring 21
      B.   Pharmacology 21
      C.   Neurotoxicology 22

V.   Performing SEP Studies 27
      A.   Experimental Design 27
      B.   Selecting the Subject 27
      C.   Preparing the Subject 27
      D.   Decisions about Stimulating and Recording 28

Acknowledgments 28

References 29

*   This manuscript has been reviewed by the Health Effects Research Laboratory U.S.E.P.A. and approved for publication. Mention of trade names or commercial products does not constitute endorsement or recommendation for use.

I. INTRODUCTION

Somatosensory evoked potentials (SEPs) have been used by neuroscientists for many years. The versatility of the method is attested to by the differing purposes to which it has been applied. Initially, SEPs were used to uncover basic principles of sensory processing. A casual glance at the literature might suggest that SEPs fell from favor and that over the last decade there has been a renaissance in their use (and the use of evoked potentials in general). More careful scrutiny indicates that use of the method has continued to increase at a steady rate, but that the arenas in which it has been used have shifted from those of basic to those of applied problems. With the advent of more advanced microelectrode techniques, SEPs were displaced from the basic neuroscience laboratory to the clinic, where they have been used by psychologists and neurologists. In turn, the apparent utility of the SEP in addressing applied problems has led to a renewed interest in some of the basic mechanisms underlying the recorded responses. The goal of the present chapter is threefold. First, to provide a critical summary of the contemporary uses of SEPs; second, to explore the potential utility of SEPs in neurotoxicology; third, to identify some of the issues which must be addressed in order to perform good neurotoxicological experiments using SEPs.

Understanding the content of this chapter will be facilitated by a simplified review of the cutaneous somatosensory pathways (proprioceptive pathways will not be discussed). Detailed discussion of the physiology and anatomy of cutaneous sensation may be found in Darian-Smith,[1] Mountcastle,[2] and Perl.[3] While the somatosensory system contains the longest axons of any sensory system, the basic layout is remarkably simple. First-order neurons have their cell bodies in the dorsal root ganglia. In the periphery, the receptors are at the ends of what appear to be long axons, although strictly speaking they are dendrites since the normal flow of activity from them is towards the first-order neuron cell body rather than away from it. Action potentials generated at the receptors are transmitted along peripheral nerves, past the cell body, into the spinal cord. It is important to note that for the most part, peripheral nerves do not segregate fibers of different sizes or types. Thus, a given peripheral nerve may contain large and small sensory fibers as well as motor fibers. Once inside the spinal cord, there are two basic somatosensory pathways: the dorsal column pathway and the spinothalamic pathway. At this point the pathway a particular fiber takes depends upon fiber size, fiber type, and nature of the sensation mediated.

Large (A alpha and A beta) fast ($\approx$100 M/sec) fibers bend rostrally upon entering the cord, and ascend in the dorsal columns or spinocervical tract to the medulla. At the medulla these fibers synapse in the dorsal column nuclei. Axons from dorsal column nucleus cells cross the midline and ascend in the medial lemniscus to the thalamus, where they form synapses largely with cells in the lateral portion of the ventrobasal complex. Axons from cells in the ventrobasal complex ascend to the somatosensory cortex, where they terminate in locations dependent upon the part of the body they represent. This dorsal column system is thought to mediate the most complex aspects of mechanoreception, including tacticle discrimination and sensory control of movement.

Small (A delta and C) slow (<30 M/sec) fibers, upon entering the spinal cord, synapse immediately in the dorsal horn, primarily in layer V, but also in layers I, IV, and VI. Axons from the second-order neurons cross to the other side of the cord, where they ascend in the spinothalamic tracts all the way to the ventrobasal complex of the thalamus. As with the dorsal column system, the third-order neurons in the spinothalamic system carry action potentials from the thalamus to the somatosensory cortex, where they too terminate in a topographic fashion related to the sensory field of origin. The spinothalamic system is presumed to mediate such course sensations as pain and temperature. These pathways are summarized in Figure 1.

Electrical stimulation of a peripheral nerve is likely to activate both the dorsal column

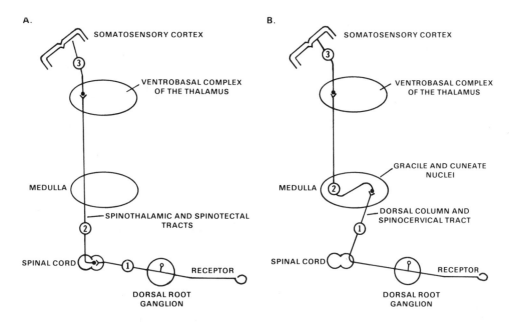

FIGURE 1. Schematic drawing of the major somatosensory pathways. (A) Spinothalamic system; (B) dorsal column system. Circled numbers indicate the neuron number in the chain. Thus, 3 indicates third-order neuron.

and spinothalamic systems, since most peripheral nerves contain a mixture of axon sizes and types. The resulting evoked potential waveform recorded at the cortical level is therefore an integrated reflection of multiple inputs. SEPs have been recorded from many noncortical levels, including the mixed peripheral nerves, various levels of the spinal cord, brainstem, and thalamus. This chapter will focus on the waveforms which may be recorded from the scalp, skull, or cortex, although as will be seen, inferences may be made about some subcortical activities from these recordings.

II. THE PHENOMENOLOGY OF SEPs

Perhaps more than any other literature on commonly recorded evoked potentials, the SEP literature is characterized by basic differences between laboratories in the morphology of the waveforms reported. The mean and range of latencies of major evoked potential peaks recorded from the scalp of humans following stimulation of the median nerve in seven different groups of subjects are illustrated in Figure 2. This plot does not reflect far-field responses (see below).

In addition to variability between studies in mean peak latencies, there is also variabilty between studies in the amount of intrastudy variability. Coefficients of variations were calculated for each peak in the studies used to construct Figure 2, and the means and ranges of these values are presented in Table 1. The table illustrates that, contrary to conventional wisdom, variability in the latency of late peaks is not much greater than variability in the latency of early peaks. The table also indicates that not all groups of subjects display all peaks.

Between-study variations in SEP waveform morphology are important for several reasons. If a waveform is to be used as a means to detect and characterize dysfunction, one must be capable of comparing types of effects across studies. For example, if one laboratory finds that toxicant A produces a 50% reduction in the amplitude of a positive wave that peaks 20 msec after the stimulus, and another study finds no effect of the closely related toxicant A', but also shows no positive peak in control animals anywhere near 20 msec, very little can

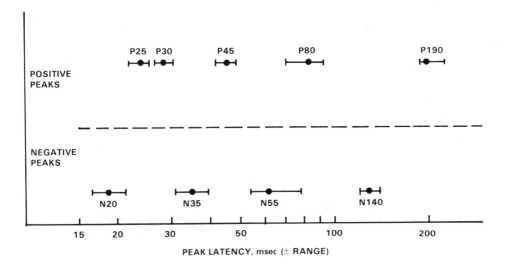

FIGURE 2.   Mean and range of latencies for major peaks of SEPs recorded from the scalp of seven different groups of human subjects. In all cases the contralateral median nerve was stimulated. The figure illustrates the extent of between study variability in SEPs.[45]

Table 1
MEDIAN NERVE SEP LATENCY COEFFICIENTS OF
VARIATION (CVs) OBTAINED IN 7 GROUPS OF
HUMANS REPORTED BY GIBLIN[45]

	Peak name			
	N20	N35	N55	N140
CV range (%)	1—10	2—14	1—11	2—12
CV mean (%)	5.57	8.29	7.4	7.7
CV SEM	1.2	1.9	1.9	3.0
Number of studies reporting this peak	7	7	5	3
	P25	P30	P45	P80
CV range (%)	0.2—17	5—14	1—16	5—12
CV mean (%)	6.0	9.75	8.29	8.25
CV SEM	3.0	2.0	2.1	1.5
Number of studies reporting this peak	5	4	7	4

be said about the relative effects of A and A' on the somatosensory system. Further, it will always be desirable to link changes in waveform properties with the underlying physiological processes. Since each study will not be able to assess the physiological processes which underlie the waveforms it reports, reliance must be made upon historical determinations, yet it is not possible to rely upon the results from previous studies if the waveforms have markedly different morphology. Therefore, some standardization of waveforms, as appears to have occurred in the visual system,[4,5] is desirable.

A. SEP Peak Nomenclature

Three strategies for labeling evoked potential (EP) peaks have been commonly employed. First, peaks may be simply numbered consecutively, I, II, III, etc. Second, peaks may be identified by their polarity and consecutive numbers, such that the first negative peak is N1, the third positive peak is P3, etc. The third strategy is to identify the peak by its polarity and approximate latency, such that if the first negative peak normally occurred between 19 and 21 msec after the stimulus, it would be designated N20. The first strategy has commonly been mixed with the others, such that early far-field positive peaks (see below) may be designated I, II, III, but that the first cortically generated positive peak may be called P1. Comparing waveforms between studies is often difficult because of these different strategies, yet there are occasions when each appears appropriate. For example, when comparing SEPs between species, it makes more sense to compare the properties of the first cortical peaks than to try to keep track of the equivalent latencies for them all. On the other hand, when comparing waveforms recorded from different loci in the same subject, it makes more sense to keep track of the latency than the peak number. For example, if a recording is obtained from the contralateral central area of humans (C4) referred to the midforehead (Fp$_z$), the first negative peak following median nerve stimulation will be at about 20 msec (N1 = N20). However, if the recording is made between the neck (e.g., C2) and Fp$_z$, the negative peak occurring 20 msec after stimulation will be the third negative peak (N3 = N20), yet the N20 peak has the same generator in both cases.[6] In this chapter an effort will be made to provide the reader with both types of information. Peaks which are clearly precortical in origin but which can be recorded from the scalp will be identified with consecutive Roman numerals, unless otherwise stated. Cortically generated peaks will be identified by polarity and peak number. If the authors have used a peak latency designation, this will be included in parentheses.

Once a waveform has achieved some standardization, it is desirable to also achieve an understanding of the generators of the waveform. Such an understanding comes at a cost of great effort, since it entails evaluating (1) the area from which the SEP is maximally recorded (which may be different for different peaks in an SEP), (2) the cortical depth of the active area (if the source is in fact in the cortex), (3) the inputs to the active areas (e.g., are they local, thalamic, commissural, etc.), and (4) whether the peak reflects predominantly excitatory or inhibitory activity.

It is not necessary that a full understanding of SEPs be achieved if the technique is to be used only as a screen. In the simplest screening case it is only necessary to know that waveforms from a treated group are similar to or different from those of a control group. However, since EP waveforms do contain information which may allow some characterization of the nature of differences from control, it makes sense to capitalize when possible. Indeed, it will be suggested below that the SEP is most useful in verifying the existence and pinpointing the locus of somatosensory dysfunction, and of questionable value for general screening.

A few published studies have described in detail attempts to determine the active areas responsible for SEPs produced in the cortex. Arezzo et al.[7] report spatiotemporal properties of SEPs evoked in macaques by electrical stimulation of the contralateral median nerve. Figures 3 to 5 illustrate some of their findings.

Figure 3 shows SEPs recorded from four epidural loci in the unanesthetized macaque. The surface distribution of the identified peaks is illustrated in Figure 4. If a common underlying circuitry was responsible for the entire waveform, all isopotential maps in Figure 4 should be identical. Clearly, they are not all identical. It is evident that, owing to unique loci for the different peaks, slight variation in electrode location can increase or decrease the amplitude of selected peaks, independent of others. This finding has important implications for neurotoxicology. Between-subjects experimental designs must take extraordinary care to ensure uniform electrode placement across subjects. Figure 5 makes the point that the sources for the various SEP peaks are cortical and not subcortical, since polarity of the response reverses as an electrode is moved through the cortex.

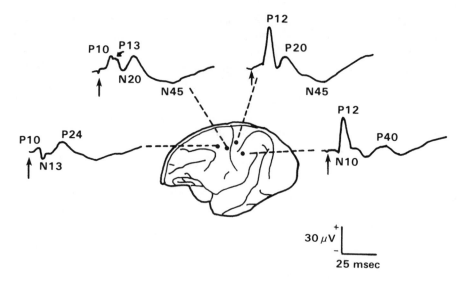

FIGURE 3.   SEPs recorded from four epidural loci in the macaque brain following electrical stimulation of the contralateral median nerve. Arrows mark the stimulus onset. Peaks are identified by polarity (P vs. N) and latency. The SEPs recorded from different loci vary in amplitude, relative prominence of peaks, and in some cases polarity of peaks.[7]

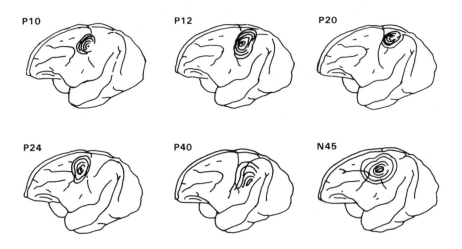

FIGURE 4.   Isopotential maps illustrating, from the surface distribution for several of the peaks identified in Figure 3, that not all of the peaks in the macaque median nerve evoked SEP are generated in the same cortical area. Areas where the amplitude recorded was greater than 90% of the maximum amplitude are darkened. Each outer line reflects progressive 10% reductions in amplitude.[7]

According to Arezzo et al.,[7] P1 (P10) and P2 (P12), the earliest cortically generated SEP components in macaques, arise in Brodmann's area 3, and Brodmann's areas 1 and 2, respectively. Both peaks are resistant to barbiturate anesthesia. The P4 (P20) peak, only present in the alert monkey, is generated in areas 2 and 5. It is noteworthy that area 5 receives multimodality input, and has been associated with complex processing of somatosensory information, and that the human "equivalent" of this peak (P40) may bear some relationship to cognitive function.[8] The P6 (P40) peak appears to arise from area 7a, while the P8 (P110) peak originates over a wide range of cortical areas, including areas 5 and 7b.

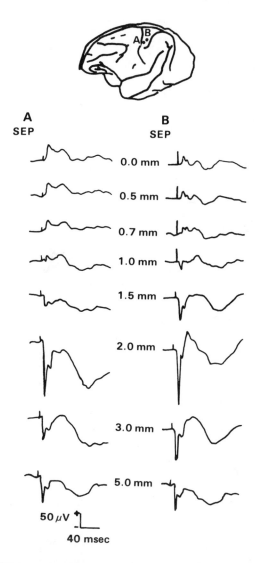

FIGURE 5. SEPs recorded from different depths within the cortex of macaques at two cortical sites, A and B. Distances listed adjacent to recordings indicate the depth from the cortical surface. Note the polarity reversal, particularly evident for the initial deflection.[7]

There appear to be good correlations between the topography of these peaks recorded from monkeys and those recorded from humans, although absolute latencies are longer in the human case.[7,9]

The Arezzo et al.[7] study represents a major step in our understanding of the various waveform morphologies recorded from the monkey, as well as the topographic location of the generators. Further steps must be taken to understand more fully the microcircuitry within the cortex responsible for locally generated peaks, including identification of the relative roles of EPSPs and IPSPs in different cell layers which generate each peak. The magnitude of the task yet to be performed may be appreciated when considering we have only discussed stimulation of the median nerve. Other commonly stimulated sites are the tibial nerve, the sural nerve, peroneal nerve, sciatic nerve, and trigeminal nerve. While stimulation of each of these sites may produce a different waveform with different topographic distribution, some principles may be emerging. For example, a recent study by Dong and Chudler[10]

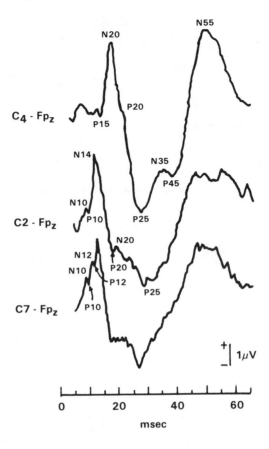

FIGURE 6.   Averaged SEPs recorded in a human following 1000 stimulations of the median nerve at the
wrist. Simultaneous recordings from the contralateral
central area (C_4) and two neck regions (C_2, C_7), all
referred to the midforehead (f_{pz}).[6]

investigated the origin of SEPs recorded in cats following toothpulp stimulation. The earliest
activity of cortical origin was a positive peak which occurred with a latency of about 6
msec, and like the human monkey cases, had its source in Brodmann's area 3.

B. Far-Field Potentials

   To this point, discussion has focused upon SEP components which reflect activity in the
cortex. The last 7 years has witnessed an explosion of interest in the small short latency
potentials which precede the cortical SEP waves. These "far-field", or short latency potentials are presumed to reflect activity volume conducted from different subcortical loci
and as such may provide a means to monitor with some precision the site of dysfunction in
the diseased or otherwise dysfunctional nervous system. Figure 6 contains examples of far-
field SEPs (FFSEPs). Note that the peaks are often inflection points which barely disturb
the rising slope of the initial cortical peak. In order to detect these tiny peaks reliably and
accurately, one must average more responses than with cortical SEPs (usually >500 responses, as compared to about 100 responses). In addition, greater care must be taken to
avoid filtering of the high frequencies which make up the FFSEP components.

   While the final word on the sources for each of the FFSEP peaks has certainly not been
written, it seems likely that the waves reflect activity of action potentials in tracts, rather
than EPSPs and IPSPs.[11] The three positive peaks occurring prior to the initial cortical

response (Nl in humans) have been described as arising from the thalamus (I), thalamocortical afferents (II), and further thalamocortical afferents (III) in rats, cats, monkeys, and humans,[12,13] or from the posterior columns of the spinal cord (I), posterior column nuclei and medical lemniscus (II), and thalamus and thalamo-cortical radiations (III) in rats.[14] The former interpretation is supported by recordings from shoulder, neck, and skull/scalp in the indicated species, while the latter is supported by direct recordings from subcortical loci as well as ability to follow stimuli of varying frequency. A comparison of peak latencies recorded from rats in the above two studies suggests that different waveforms may have been recorded, since the response Wiederholt and Iragui-Madoz[14] report as I occurred at a peak of about 2.01 msec after the stimulus, while the apparently same peak (from inspection of the figures) in the Allison et al.[13] study had a latency of 4.9 msec. The difference is probably not accounted for by the fact that Allison et al.[13] used a stimulus intensity just sufficient to produce a finger movement while Wiederholt and Iragui-Madoz[14] used an intensity sufficient to produce a maximal amplitude P1, since the P1 latencies reported in the two studies were quite similar, 7.5 and 7.0 msec, respectively. If stimulus intensity accounted for the differences, then the cortical response should have been more delayed in the Allison et al.[13] study than the 0.5 msec indicated. Differences in recording electrode placement may account for the different morphologies.

Arezzo et al.[15] have pointed out some of the difficulties in identifying sources of FFSEP peaks. First, since, by definition, far-field potentials are widely recorded, selection of an "indifferent" reference electrode is problematic. The optimal location for the reference electrode must be based not only on distance from the source, but also on a knowledge of the presumed geometry of the source. In particular, Arezzo et al.[15] recommend that for stimulation of the median nerve an appropriate reference site is the contralateral wrist, which happens to lie in a direction perpendicular to the rostro-caudal axis of maximum field potentials produced by the stimulus.

Second, Arezzo et al.[15] caution against inferring sources based solely on appropriate latencies of potentials recorded from a particular candidate locus. The candidate locus may have a geometry which makes generation of far-field potentials unlikely. For example, the ventrobasal complex of the thalamus and the dorsal column nuclei appear to have a "closed field" geometry, which would minimize spread of postsynaptic potentials. The potentials generated at this putative source may merely overlap in time with potentials generated more caudally. Thus, unequivocal identification of a source requires stepwise tracing of the potential from its maximum to the location from which recordings are normally made. From these considerations it is evident that further analysis of the interpretation of Wiederholt and Iragui-Madoz[14] and Allison et al.[13] may be in order. Recent intracranial recordings from humans have made a compelling case that the three most prominent far-field waves recorded from scalp loci: I (P9), II (P11), and III (P14), derive from peripheral nerve, cervical dorsal column, and medial lemniscus, respectively.[16,17]

The brainstem auditory evoked response (BAER) was the first far-field potential to achieve wide acceptance as a clinical measure.[18] An appealing characteristic of the BAER is that subtracting the latency to the first peak from the latency to the last peak provides what has been called "central conduction time". Central conduction time is not affected by alterations in the periphery, since these would be constant at the first and last peak of the response. Therefore, the measure provides an index of the integrity of function within the brainstem. A similar measure has been developed and is becoming popular in the somatosensory system.

In the somatosensory system the most common technique for determining central conduction time has been to obtain separate recordings from the neck and scalp following stimulation of either the median or peroneal nerve.[6,19,20] When the human median nerve is stimulated, the measure of central conduction time is given by N20-N14, where N20 is presumed to reflect the first cortically generated peak and N14 is presumed to arise from the dorsal columns in the cervical cord.

C. Species Comparisons

As with any end-point under consideration for use in assessing toxicity, it is important to evaluate generality across species. One of the major advantages of sensory evoked potentials (not just SEPs) is that they may be recorded noninvasively from humans, thereby raising the prospect of a very direct extrapolation from laboratory animal to human. In order to capitalize upon this prospect, one must establish the analogies and homologies between waveforms recorded from humans and various species of laboratory animal. Having done so, it may be possible to use species like the rat for screening and early characterization purposes, while reserving more expensive species like monkeys for selected cases.

In drawing comparisons between waveforms recorded from different species, three constraints should be considered. First, and perhaps most obvious, is that absolute latency is not a useful cross-species comparison variable. Latency is directly related to length of the pathway, and inversely related to diameter of the stimulated fibers. While an approximate length of the pathway may be determined noninvasively with a tape measure, diameter of the stimulated fibers may not. Small animals like the rat have shorter pathways than humans, thereby decreasing SEP latencies. However, the rat also has small-diameter fibers, thereby increasing SEP latencies. Consequently, initial comparisons between species are most sensibly made on a peak number rather than a peak latency basis (e.g., first peak, second peak, etc.).

Second, one cannot assume *a priori* that the synaptic inputs to homologous brain regions are the same. In a hypothetical case, the first positive peak recorded from one brain region in the monkey might reflect locally generated activity, while the homologous peak in a rat may reflect volume conducted activity from a nearby cortical area. The peaks are homologous but not analogous. In view of this possibility, direct comparisons between species are inappropriate until some evidence exists that the comparison peaks have common determinants (are analogous). If such comparisons are to be made despite their inappropriateness, peak number should be used for the description. The underlying principle is that in the absence of analogy, homology is better than chaos.

The validity of cross-species FFSEP comparisons has been addressed by Allison and Hume[12] and Allison et al.[13] Allison and Hume[12] performed surface and depth recordings in monkeys and cats, comparing their findings to surface recordings from monkeys, cats, rats, and humans. All stimuli were applied to the median nerve at the wrist, with intensity just sufficient to elicit a twitch in the first digit. For recordings intended to reflect cortical activity, the reference was placed either in the frontal bone or in the overlying scalp. Active electrodes were placed over contralateral parietal areas, although it is not clear what criteria were used for this placement in cats and rats.

Initial cortically generated activity was a positive wave in rats and cats, but a negative wave in humans in monkeys. Nevertheless, depth recordings provided evidence that these reflected similar generators. The mean latencies of this first cortical peak were 19.2, 12.0, 11.3, and 7.5 msec for humans, monkeys, cats, and rats, respectively.[13] The between-species surface polarity difference is presumed to reflect the presence of a complex gyral pattern in primates. Figure 7 shows schematically the relative latencies of peaks between species, and Table 2 shows the actual latencies recorded.

As suggested above, the presence and nature of gyri near the recording electrode can produce drastic between-species alterations in surface topography of recorded potentials. An example of how such changes might occur may be seen in Figure 8.

It would appear that matters would be simplest in the lissencephalic brains of such animals as rats. While this may be true theoretically, the absence of gyri presents special problems of its own. In primates and carnivores, the boundaries of many cytoarchitectonic fields may be approximated or even defined by the gyral pattern. For example, the primary somatosensory cortex, generally recognized as Brodmann's area 3, is considered to be on the postcentral gyrus of humans and postcentral gyrus of macaques. Raccoons appears to have

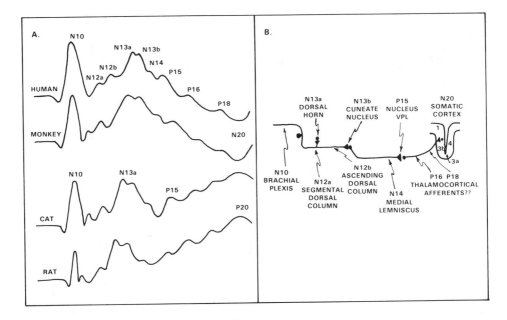

FIGURE 7. (A) Scheme showing relative latencies of human and animal early SEP components. For comparison, the peaks corresponding to the human N10 and N20/P20 are aligned with the human peaks, and other components in the animals are drawn proportionally. Each waveform is a composite of features recorded from different loci. (B) Scheme illustrating one view, based on recording from animals, of the primary generators of each component.[13]

Table 2
MEAN (± SD) PEAK LATENCY OF SEP COMPONENTS IN MAN, MONKEY, CAT, AND RAT[13]

	Human (N = 93)	Monkey (N = 5)	Cat (N = 9)	Rat (N = 6)
N10	10.1 (0.9)	5.3 (1.2)	2.8 (0.3)	1.5 (0.2)
N12a	11.6 (1.1)	5.9 (1.2)	3.6 (0.4)	1.7 (0.1)
N12b	12.2 (1.1)	6.4 (1.2)	4.2 (0.4)	2.5 (0.4)
N13a	13.5 (1.1)	7.5 (1.5)	5.4 (0.4)	3.0 (0.3)
N13b	13.8 (1.2)	8.0 (1.5)	5.8 (0.4)	3.4 (0.4)
N14	14.4 (1.1)	8.7 (1.6)	6.6 (0.5)	4.0 (0.5)
P15	15.1 (1.1)	9.3 (1.7)	7.7 (0.6)	4.9 (0.5)
P16	16.6 (1.1)	10.4 (1.8)	9.0 (0.5)	5.7 (0.5)
P18	18.3 (1.1)	11.3 (1.9)	10.2 (0.7)	6.6 (0.5)
N20/P20	19.2 (1.2)	12.0 (2.0)	11.3 (0.7)	7.5 (0.5)

an individual sensory gyrus for each finger and volar area of the paw.[21] In rats there are virtually no surface landmarks to be used, although some have attempted to relate vascular patterns to underlying brain area.[22] A recent effort, which mapped the secondary somatosensory area of the rat forepaw, attempted to use skull landmarks.[23] The authors reported that while the target area was about 0.5 mm in diameter, its location with respect to skull landmarks varied from rat to rat by as much as several millimeters. What these findings suggest is that while one is less likely to be fooled by surface topography-related polarity inversions in the rat, one is more likely to have difficulty reproducing from one rat to the next the optimal recording site. Or, put differently, a recording site determined *a priori*

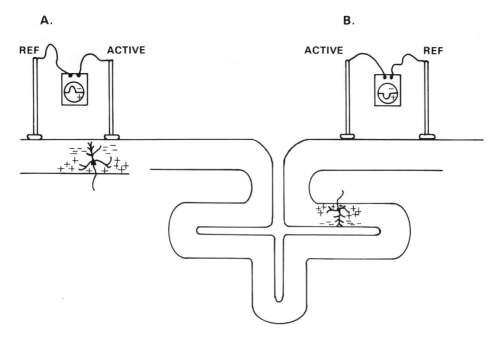

FIGURE 8.   Simple example illustrating how the presence of gyri can distort potentials recorded from the surface. (A) The undistorted case; (B) potential inversion produced by the presence of gyri.

according to skull surface landmarks, as is likely to be the case in chronic studies,[24,25] is likely to produce data with significant between animal variability.

These caveats not withstanding, some information regarding the presumed location of somatosensory cortex in rats will be provided. Figures 9 and 10 are maps which reflect the cortical distribution of single units reponsive to stimulation of different regions of the body in anesthetized rats.[26,27]

It is unfortunate that neither map shows a representation of the tail, since the tail contains the most accessible nerves for stimulation in rodents.[24,25,28,29] It is also evident from the figures that the head region is afforded by far the most expansive cortical representation. Indeed, Welker[22] estimated that while the entire trunk and tail of the rat was represented by about 7% of the primary somatosensory cortex (SmI), the vibrissae, head, and neck region was represented by over 66% of SmI. Investigators interested in using SEPs to study the rat somatosensory system could profitably attend to this anatomical convenience, but none have yet done so.

Only one paper was found which attempted to plot in a systematic way rat SEP amplitude as a function of skull location.[30] In this case the primary interest was in comparing the distribution of what is probably a P2 response as a function of type of stimulus to the hindleg. However, the absence of any comparative identification of this peak with other peaks in the literature, despite the fact that it is shown to reverse polarity in the cortex, diminishes its contribution.

There have been sufficiently few rat SEP papers that it is possible to display a good percentage of them in Figure 11. This figure shows waveforms redrawn from several studies on rats. From this figure it may be seen that significant cortical activity follows the initial P1 response in most cases, but only rarely did the papers attend to these later peaks. Table 3 provides information on the recording and stimulating loci for the waveforms depicted in Figure 11.

While the difficulties associated with recording from the lissencephalic brains of animals with only minimal cortical representation of limbs may account in part for the relatively

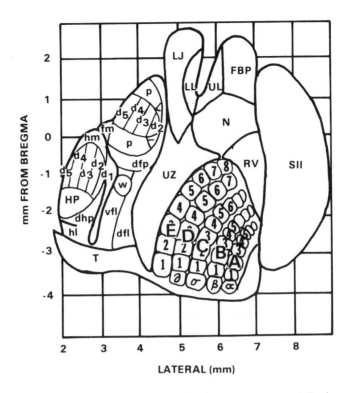

FIGURE 9.   Composite map illustrating the cutaneous representation in the primary somatosensory cortex of the anesthetized rat, determined by microelectrode mapping. Abbreviations: T, trunk; hl, hindlimb; HP, hindpaw; dhp, dorsal hindpaw; d1-5, digits 1-5 of hindpaw; hm, hindlimb muscle; vfl, ventral forelimb; dfl, dorsal forelimb; w, wrist whiskers; dfp, dorsal forepaw; p, palm; d2-5, digits 2-5 of forepaw; t, thumb; UZ, unresponsive zone; A-E, 1-8, rows (from dorsal to ventral) and numbers (from caudal to rostral) of mystacial vibrissae; RV rostral small vibrissae; N, nose; FBP, frontobuccal pads; UL, upper lip; LL, lower lip; LJ, lower jaw; SII, secondary somatosensory cortex.[26]

meagre output of rat SEP papers, neurotoxicologists should be quick to recognize the value in using this economical species. The aforementioned concerns are much less compelling in the case of FFSEPs, since they are widely distributed across the skull, and it may be that this waveform will be of significant use to neurotoxicologists.

D. Development of the SEP

Charting the developmental course by which an evoked potential reaches its adult configuration should provide clues to the stage of development of the underlying neuronal processes. Alterations in the development of a waveform produced by a toxicant may in turn be used to infer abnormal development of the nervous system. Detailed and contemporary studies of the development of SEPs in nonhuman species are rare. However several careful studies in humans, describing developmental changes at both ends of the age spectrum, provide useful information.

In the young of many species, including newborn kitten,[31] premature sheep,[32] rabbit,[33] and premature baboon,[34] the first poststimulus (median nerve) sign of cortical activity is a surface negative wave. It has been presumed that this wave corresponds to the N1(N22) wave in humans.[35] In humans, the amplitude of N1 does not change between 3 months and young adulthood, but its duration gradually decreases during this time.[35] In adult members of nonhuman species, with the exception of macaques, the first poststimulus sign of activity

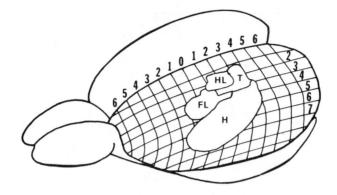

FIGURE 10.   Map of somatosensory cortex in the rat in proportion to the cerebral hemisphere, and based upon single or multiple unit responses to light tactile stimuli recorded from 16 rats. FL, foreleg; HL, hindleg; T, truck; H, head.[27]

Table 3
RECORDING CONFIGURATIONS FOR RAT SEPs IN FIGURE 11

Figure 11 Section	Stim locus	Rat strain	Coordinates re: bregma (AP/Lat) Active	Ref.	Pl Latency (msec)	Ref.
A	Forepaw	S-D	+1, +2/3,4	Nasal bone	7.23	63
B	Forepaw	S-D	+1/3.5	Post. cortex	5.75	87
C	Forepaw	S-D	~+1/~4.5	~+16/0?	7.0	14
G	Hindpaw	S-D	~+1/~2.5	~+16/0?	~11.5	14
H	Hindpaw	S-D	0/2	~+30/0?	10.75	109
I	Hindleg	L-E	−2/2.5	−8/3	~50[a]	30
E	Tail	L-E	+2/2	−4/3	23.3	116
D	Tail	L-E	−2.5/2.5	+2/2	23[b]	24
F	Tail	F-344	−2/2	Nasal bone	27.5[c]	25

[a]   Labeled P1, but probably P2.
[b]   Labeled P2, but probably P1.
[c]   Unlabeled, but probably P1.

recorded from the cortex is positive, not negative. It has been presumed that differential maturation of apical and basal dendrites converts the negative wave into a positive wave in older animals,[35] and that therefore N1 in adult monkeys and humans is functionally equivalent to P1 in other species.[13] In fact, it is not known that the negative wave which appears around birth in many species does correspond to N1 in humans, nor is it known that it is this same wave which changes polarity to become P1 with progressive development or whether the same sequence of events pertains to all these species. For example, stimulation of the tibial nerve produces a surface-negative wave in newborn rats,[36] and while several studies have shown that this surface-negative wave is retained, it appears that a surface positive wave may emerge at an earlier poststimulus time during the third postnatal week.[37,38]

The apparent correspondence between the human and monkey N1 on the one hand, and, for example, the cat P1 on the other, makes determination of the origin of the transient N1 in nonprimates of some interest.[12] In aged humans the amplitude of N1 increases, a phenomenon which is accompanied by but not highly correlated with an increased duration of the wave.[39] No studies of SEPs in aged nonhuman species were found, but it would be of

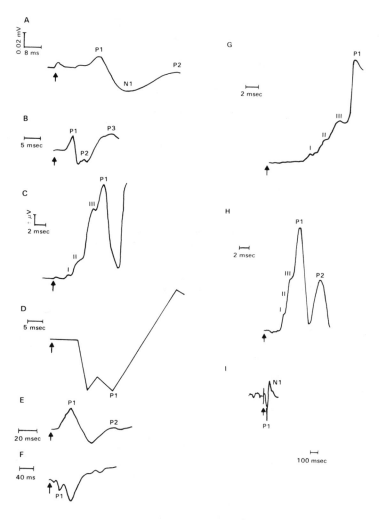

FIGURE 11. Composite figure showing SEPs recorded in rats from various loci. Details are indicated in Table 3.

interest to learn whether an early negative wave reappears in aged nonhuman species, or whether any other waves change with age in a manner that parallels the changes in the human N1.

A simple analysis of the onset latency of the N1 peak in humans reveals strikingly little change across the first 8 years of life. However, latency is subject to misinterpretation in developmental SEP studies. Pathways become longer until adulthood, thereby producing increases in latency. In order to make a rough correction for growth, the latency has been divided by the body size, to produce a millisecond per meter value. Note that this body size/factor is constant for an individual regardless of which nerve is stimulated. The value obtained should not be confused with the reciprocal of conduction velocity, in which the unit of length is specific to the nerve under test. When plotted this way (see Figure 12), a power function indicates the development of the system.[39] This trend reverses in aged humans, such that N1 latency becomes gradually longer between ages 18 and 95.[40] At least some of this increase is evidently due to slowed central conduction time in older subjects.[41]

The first positive peak of cortical origin in humans, P1, develops its adult latency at about the same rate as N1,[35,40] but increases from early adulthood to old age more rapidly than

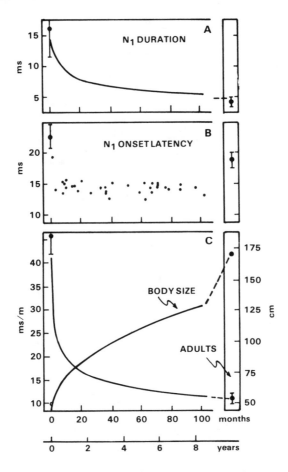

FIGURE 12.   Pooled data on N1 duration and N1 onset latency in humans, as a function of age and body size. (A) N1 duration in msec, with curve drawn according to a calculated power function. (B) N1 onset latency in milliseconds. (C) Ascending function, change in body size with age; descending function, onset latency divided by body length in milliseconds per meter, with curve drawn according to a calculated power function.[35]

does N1, thereby suggesting (1) separate generators and (2) more rapid aging of one generator than another.[40,41] In contrast to N1, P1 appears to grow in amplitude throughout life.[35,39] This differential shift in peaks with age may be responsible for the higher incidence of the "W" waveform (as described by Giblin[45]) in elderly than young adults.[39]

E. Gender Differences in SEPs

It is a common observation in the evoked potential literature that there are significant gender differences,[42] and it is therefore not surprising to find such differences with SEPs. As with visual evoked potentials, SEPs of human females are greater in amplitude than those of males.[43] Latency differences between genders have also been found, with males tending to have somewhat longer latencies. Evidently only part of these differences may be attributed to body size.[40,43]

The preceding sections have described the phenomenology of SEPs, focusing upon where they come from and what they look like. An underlying assumption is that analysis of SEPs may tell us something about the integrity of somatic sensation and the somatosensory system on one hand, and the integrity of brain function in a more general sense on the other. In the following section some of the interpretations which have been applied to alterations in SEPs will be discussed.

II. INTERPRETATION OF SEPs

A. Relationship of SEPs to Perception

While there is little need to doubt a relationship between SEPs and the perception of somatic sensation, there have been only a few attempts to explore the nature of the relationship. Soininen and Jarvilehto[44] have demonstrated in humans that reliable SEPs could be recorded at the detection threshold for tactile stimulation, but not below. The authors described a series of positive and negative peaks following threshold stimulation, but the waveform reported is not easily compared to other published waveforms since most other studies have used stimuli so great that latencies would be considerably shorter and amplitudes considerably larger. Further, use of natural (mechanical) stimulation instead of the more traditional electrical stimulation would not be expected to activate the large, fast-conducting muscle and joint afferents mediating proprioception. Consequently the neuronal activity present in many SEP studies was not present in the Soininen and Jarvilehto[44] study. These unusual characteristics of the study permitted some remarkable findings. The recorded waveforms were not simply a reflection of stimulus amplitude, since on some trials a stimulus with a particular intensity was detected while on other trials a stimulus of the same intensity was not detected. When the detected trials were averaged, an SEP was present, but when the undetected trials with the same intensity stimulus were averaged, an SEP was not observed. In other words, presence of the waveform was associated more with sensation than with the physical properties of the stimulus.

SEPs recorded following electrical stimulation of a mixed nerve such as the median nerve may largely reflect the integrity of the sense of joint position, since this sense is carried by the largest and fastest fibers. The Soininen and Jarvilehto[44] study demonstrates that, under appropriate conditions, SEP amplitude reflects light tactile sensation. It is difficult to test the integrity of the pain and temperature senses in mixed nerves since fibers which carry pain and temperature information have high thresholds and are slowly conducting. Indeed, clinical studies have indicated that humans with inability to experience pain and temperature due to spinal cord lesions may have normal SEPs.[45]

Nevertheless, there are SEP paradigms which may be useful for assessment of pain as well. A delta and C fibers are presumed to mediate the sensation of pain. Since the tooth pulp contains primarily A delta and C fibers,[46] electrical stimulation of the tooth pulp has been used as a model system for studies of pain. In this context, SEPs evoked following tooth pulp stimulation have been investigated as objective measures of pain. The SEP recorded from the vertex following tooth pulp stimulation is composed of three negative peaks and two positive peaks. The latencies of these peaks vary with the study, but N1 normally appears between 60 and 80 msec, P1 between 80 and 140 msec, N2 between 175 and 260 msec, and P2 between 260 and 400 msec.[47,48] While it is not clear whether there is a relationship between the presence and absence of pain reports and the presence and absence of SEPs at perithreshold levels of stimulation, it has been demonstrated that there is a good linear correlation between SEP amplitude and magnitude of the reported painful sensation.[47,48] In these studies, amplitude of the later peaks (N2P2 and P2N3) correlated more highly than did amplitude of the early peaks with pain magnitude. Administration of a placebo reduces both the N2P2 amplitude and the reported magnitude of pain, implying that sensation is more potent than stimulus magnitude as a determinant of SEP amplitude.[49]

From the above studies and others[50] it might appear that amplitude of SEPs evoked by electrical stimulation would correlate with proprioceptive sensation. While this is a difficult assumption to test, some data suggest that is it not entirely accurate. Schiff et al.[51] have recorded SEPs from a population of patients with focal disease of the spinal cord which included some with proprioceptive deficit. While it was true that most of the patients with a proprioceptive deficit had abnormal SEPs, it was also true that many patients without disordered proprioception had disordered SEPs. Only latencies were evaluated, and a direct test of the hypothesis is therefore not possible, but it is noteworthy that one patient had apparently normal proprioception but an absent scalp response to peroneal nerve stimulation.

The underlying principle of interpretation to be learned from these studies is that amplitude of the SEP may be correlated with magnitude of sensation, as long as care is taken to study only the sensation mediated by the largest and fastest fibers likely to be activated by the stimulus. It is also important to note the possibility that while such relationships may exist in the normal brain, the correlations may break down under conditions of disease or neurotoxic insult.

B. SEP Changes in Neurological Disorders

Various investigators have reported SEP changes in patients with neurological disorders ranging from focal peripheral lesions to diffuse and global cerebral dysfunction. While it may not be reasonable to expect wholesale parallels between findings reported in the neurological clinic and those obtained in the neurotoxicology laboratory, awareness of the kinds of abnormalities observed in patients with known or presumed neurological disease may aid neurotoxicologists to interpret their own findings.

As would be expected, peripheral nerve lesions produce abnormalities in SEPs recorded from the scalp. Typically, SEP amplitudes are greatly diminished and latencies are increased, both in rough proportion to the extent of damage. Occasionally, these changes precede clinically detectable sensory dysfunction. When a focal disorder such as carpal tunnel syndrome is present, the waveform morphology is relatively normal, but shifted in latency. Other peripheral nerve disorders may produce gross waveform distortion.[45]

Spinal cord lesions produce effects upon SEPs which seem to be partially dependent upon location of the lesion. Lesions in humans involving the dorsal column system may abolish SEPs, while anterolateral tractotomy may leave them unaffected.[45] Demyelinating disease produces increased latencies, even in some cases when no clinical deficit in joint position sense has been detected.[52]

It should be noted that in most cases in which electrical stimulation has been used, a stimulus intensity is chosen which is either near threshold intensity or at a small multiple (usually 2) of the threshold intensity required to produce a motor response. Use of these stimulus intensities may account for the failure to detect from SEPs any alterations in pathways carrying higher threshold pain and temperature information. Powers et al.[53] used high-intensity (20 times the motor threshold) stimulation of the posterior tibial nerve in a series of cats with nine different combinations of unilateral spinal cord lesions. The cats were anesthetized with a ketamine xylazine mixture. Immediately after motor threshold was determined, they were paralyzed to avoid the recording difficulties associated with movement and muscle artifacts.

Figure 13 illustrates the altered waveform morphology produced by higher-intensity stimulation. Several late negative peaks are evident in the records following high-intensity stimulation which are not present in the records following threshold stimulation. Lesions in the dorsal columns resulted in severe attenuation of amplitudes of early (P1N2) and late (N4) peaks measured from the side of the brain ipsilateral to the lesion. Lesions of the ventrolateral tracts resulted in moderate attenuation of early and late ipsilateral peaks and severe attenuation of late contralateral peaks. Lesions of the dorsal spinocerebellar tracts resulted in severe attenuation of the early ipsilateral peaks. One may conclude from this study that with sufficiently intense stimulation an accurate picture of the integrity of the major ascending spinal cord tracts may be obtained from SEPs. High-intensity stimulation is not practical under most circumstances because it is painful and may produce large

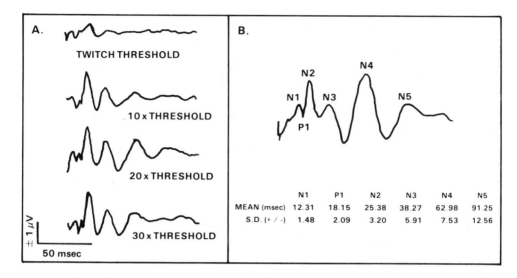

FIGURE 13.   SEPs recorded from cats, showing the effect of increasing stimulus intensity beyond twitch threshold. (A) Effects of stimulus intensity (stimuli presented at posterior tibial nerve). (B) One cat's SEP at 20 × motor threshold. Values shown in the table are mean peak latencies and standard deviations based upon 14 cats.[53]

movement artifacts, but it may be useful in neurosurgery because the subjects are anesthesized and often paralyzed as well.

When damage occurs at subcortical levels, and conventional stimulation and recording configurations are employed, the preceding summary indicates that the typical finding is either an increased latency and/or decreased amplitude of N1 (or P1), the first cortical peak. Other later peaks are generally shifted and decreased as well.[54]

When the damage is cortical, more complex patterns of change are observed, and in some cases the pattern of change may aid in localization of the lesion. In a series of 30 patients, Stohr et al.[55] found that SEP abnormalities could be divided into four types, each of which was associated with a different type of lesions. The type 1 SEP, characterized by abnormalities at all points beyond the last far-field response recorded with a frontal reference (a positive peak at 15 msec), reflected lesions of the thalamus, internal capsule and centrum semiovale. Severe attenuation of N1 (N20) and subsequent components defined a type 2 SEP, and those were associated with lesions of the postcentral gyrus. When N1 was spared but later waves lost, damage was presumed to be in parietal association areas and the response was designated a type 3 SEP. A type 4 SEP was rare. In this case, damage was in area 39, and only peaks N3 (N55) and beyond were affected. These findings generally parallel what would be expected based upon the report of Arezzo et al.[7] in monkeys.

Mauguiere et al.[56] correlated median nerve evoked SEPs with a detailed clinical examination and computerized tomographic scanning in a series of 22 patients with single circumscribed hemisphere lesions outside the basal ganglia. Responses were compared to those obtained from the unaffected hemisphere. While the onset latency of N1 (N20) recorded from scalp overlying parietal cortex was normal in these cases, the peak latency was delayed about 5% (1.1 msec). Small lesions of the postcentral gyrus which preserved tactile and deep sensation were sufficient to produce astereognosis and to reduce or eliminate N1 and P1. Similarly, Obeso et al.[57] demonstrated that focal lesions restricted to primary somatosensory cortex produced increased latency of N1 (N22) recorded from the affected side in 90% of cases, and decreased N1 amplitude almost as often (81%). Changes detected in N2 (N39) and N3 (N70) were of similar character, but were observed in fewer cases.

It might seem that increased latency and decreased amplitude are the only possible outcomes of EP studies in the presence of neurological damage. However, enhanced SEP amplitudes have been reported to follow several types of dysfunction. For example, Mauguiere et al.[56] observed that a response (P22-N30) which can be recorded from precentral gyrus (motor cortex) following median nerve stimulation was actually enhanced when parietal lesions were present. Obeso et al.[57] found that focal cortical damage remote from the recording site tended to produce increased amplitudes. For example, in patients with a unilateral lesion involving primary sensorimotor cortex, SEP N1 (N22) amplitudes recorded from the intact (contralateral) hemisphere were larger than those in control subjects 33% of the time, and smaller in less than 10% of the cases. Further, when the lesion was ipsilateral to the recording site but distant from it (i.e., in frontal, temporal, or occipital lobes), SEP N1 (N22) amplitudes were increased in 80% of cases, and decreased in the other 20%. Surprisingly, N1 (N22) and N2 (N39) were more often affected than N3 (N70). Intuitively, one might suppose that distant damage would have a more potent influence on late rather than early peaks.

Other studies have demonstrated selective enhancement of later SEP components. For example, some patients with Down's Syndrome have large late SEP components.[58] In a study involving *Macaca speciosa* monkeys, Watson et al.[59] demonstrated that a unilateral lesion in the frontal arcuate cortex had no effect upon N1 (N13), but increased latency and amplitude of P3 (P100). This same lesion produced the unilateral neglect phenomenon. While these findings are of interest, their interpretation must be tempered with the knowledge that only three monkeys were involved, and there may have been prelesion differences between the side of the brain on which lesions were ultimately made and the contralateral side, which was used as the control.

In cats, kindling of the cortex results in enhanced amplitudes of N2P3N3 following stimulation of the forepaw.[60] These enhanced SEPs may have determinants which are similar to those of the giant SEPs observed in humans with certain types of epilepsy and cortical myoclonus.[61] In the latter cases, N1 is usually not changed, but N2 is grossly enlarged. While these giant potentials are evidently not related directly to movement, they may reflect either hypersynchrony in cortical neurons, or an abnormally large input from slower conducting neurons.[62] Similarly, Takahashi and Straschill[63] report that an epileptic focus generated in rats by topical application of penicillin alters SEPs. Following forepaw stimulation, P1 (P7) and N1 (N9) amplitudes were unchanged, but P2 (P13) and N2 (N22) amplitudes were grossly enhanced.

There appear to be a number of reasons why an SEP could be abnormally large. From the preceding it is tempting to conclude that either distant or diffuse cortical damage is likely to increase the amplitude of SEPs. While this conclusion may have some validity, several studies indicate that its generality is limited. Huntington's disease has been associated with increased latency of N1 and depressed amplitudes in later SEP peaks evoked by median nerve stimulation in one study of 21 patients.[64] In another study, 32 patients with Huntington's disease were compared to 30 controls and 41 individuals at risk for Huntington's disease. In this study, latencies were not increased, but amplitudes of N1 and P1 were decreased following both median and tibial nerve stimulation.[65] While procedural differences probably account for the differences between the two studies, it is noteworthy that in both cases amplitudes were decreased.

To summarize, changes in SEPs recorded from subjects with known neurological disorders have provided added clues to aid interpretation of SEPs altered by other means. Damage which is in the subcortical somatosensory pathway tends to increase latency and decrease amplitude of far- and near-field SEPs recorded from the scalp. However, without proper stimulating conditions, damage to slowly conducting pathways may be missed. Cortical damage may increase or decrease the amplitude of SEP peaks generated in the cortex, depending upon the locus and nature of damage. Increased amplitudes may reflect distant/ diffuse damage, but all distant/diffuse damage need not be reflected in increased amplitudes.

IV. USES OF SEPs

A. Diagnosis and Surgical Monitoring

Because of variability in the SEPs recorded from normal subjects, it may never be possible to utilize a particular type of SEP abnormality in and of itself as diagnostic of a particular neurological disease. On the other hand, SEPs can and have been useful diagnostic aids for differentiating between disease states. Neurologists have looked to EPs for aid in diagnosis of multiple sclerosis (MS). While most studies which have compared the relative value of different EP techniques in recognizing MS have concluded that visual evoked potentials are most useful, it is commonly conceded that SEPs (and brainstem auditory evoked potentials) are valuable adjuncts.[66-69] It has been noted that under conditions of fever or experimental hyperthermia, differences between MS and control patients are enhanced. While increased temperature speeds conduction in the normal nervous system, it has the opposite effect upon those with definite MS.[70,71] SEPs are also altered (increased latency) in cases of amyotrophic lateral sclerosis,[72] although these patients have not been evaluated under conditions of hyperthermia.

It is known that with advanced age, SEP latencies and amplitudes increase. When these normal aging changes are taken into account there are no differences between normal subjects and patients with senile dementia of the Alzheimer type. On the other hand, patients with multi-infarct dementia have increased N1 (N20) latency, increased central conduction time, and decreased amplitude compared to Alzheimer patients. Therefore, SEPs may aid in discriminating these populations.[73]

In comatose patients there is an increased central conduction time, and occasional disintegration of SEP waves.[74] Recovery of SEP peaks appears to correlate well with recovery of the patient.[75-77] Similarly, Goff et al.[78] found that cases of Reye's syndrome, which usually is accompanied by cerebral edema, are generally associated with marked depression of all SEP components. Recovery of early components was associated with survival, and recovery of components normally occurring with latencies greater than 100 msec tended to predict that there would be no lasting neuropsychological deficit.

Use of SEPs for continuous monitoring of the integrity of somatosensory pathways has become a routine procedure.[79-81] In one recently described application,[82] SEPs were used to determine in a direct way the advisability of a particular surgical procedure for each patient. Evaluating the integrity of SEPs during carotid endartectomy allowed the surgeon to decide whether collateral circulation was adequate, and thereby determine which patients could endure the procedure without a temporary by-pass shunt to prevent ischemic brain damage during surgery.

B. Pharmacology

Anesthesia is at once the most common and heavy handed pharmacological manipulation performed in conjunction with SEP studies. In general, these studies indicate that SEP peak sensitivity to anesthesia is correlated with peak latency.[83] Allison and Hume[12] have shown that in cats, rats, and monkeys, terminal pentobarbital anesthesia results in retrogressive loss of SEP peaks, from the latest (cortical) to the earliest (far-field). In a human study in which specific peaks were not identified, it was indicated that ulnar nerve SEP alterations depended upon the anesthetic used.[84] In particular, 80% nitrous oxide severely attenuated all late SEP peaks, as did 2% diethyl ether. The entire cortically generated SEP was obliterated by 4% diethyl ether. By contrast, ethrane, a halogenated ether, produced marked increases in SEP amplitude at high concentrations (3%). Pathak et al.[85] report that fentanyl anesthesia (in the presence of 60% nitrous oxide, secobarbital, and atropine) increased all peak latencies, depressed N1P2, and increased the P2N2 amplitude of tibial nerve evoked SEPs. Ganes and Lundar[86] recorded SEPs in already comatose patients administered thiopentone, and showed that central conduction time was not altered by the anesthetic, but that all peaks beyond N1(N20) were missing.

Angel et al.[87] used forepaw stimulation SEPs in rats to study the interaction between anesthetic (urethane) requirements and changes in atmospheric pressure. In this case, SEP changes were correlated with changes in the behavioral response to tail shock. Increasing atmospheric pressure produced a linear increase in the anesthetic dose required to maintain a fixed-size behavioral response to tail shock. Similarly, increasing atmospheric pressure produced a linear increase in N1 amplitude. When atmospheric pressure was kept constant and urethane dose was increased, N1 amplitude decreased in a fashion which was nearly linear with log dose. From this study one may conclude that monitoring the amplitude of N1 in rats provided a useful measure of depth of anesthesia.

In many studies, the influence of anesthetics on SEPs is intimately tied to the influence of anesthetics on body temperature. Altered body temperature produces altered evoked potentials, and may interact with anesthesia to produce unique alterations in EP characteristics.[88,89] It is difficult to perform studies in which body temperature is systematically manipulated in the absence of anesthesia. Several studies have recorded SEPs from humans with body temperatures raised either artificially[71] or by fever of extracerebral origin.[70] In both cases, a slight increase in peripheral conduction velocity was reported in the absence of any changes in central conduction time. No changes in amplitude were reported. The temperature range over which these studies were performed (1 to 2°C elevation) and the absence of information regarding the relationship between brain temperature and body temperature under these conditions limit their generality.

In human studies in which hypothermia was achieved while the subject was anesthetized with fentanyl and nitrous oxide, peak latencies increased in a manner which was inversely proportional to temperature. Later peaks were affected more than early peaks.[82,90] Amplitude of cortically generated peaks following median nerve stimulation decreased with progressive hypothermia, but amplitude of one peripherally generated peak (N14), presumed to reflect activity in the dorsal columns, increased by 50% between 33 and 26°C.[82] In cats anesthetized with pentobarbital, hyperthermia resulted in decreased latency and increased amplitude as temperature rose to about 41°C. Beyond this point, latencies increased and amplitudes decreased.[92]

The results of Budnick et al.[92] in rats anesthetized with sodium pentobarbital essentially parallel those of Markand et al.[82] in humans. The later the normal latency of a peak, the more it was influenced by hypothermia. In general, amplitudes declined with progressive hypothermia, with the exception of component I of the FFSEP, which probably reflects dorsal column activity and which increased in amplitude between 37 and 24°C. These results are quite different from those recorded from the visual system of anesthetized rats, where combined hypothermia and anesthesia produce an increase in N1 amplitude (the first cortically generated peak), in addition to an increase in all peak latencies.[88,89]

While a number of studies have investigated the role of various neurotransmitters in the functioning of somatosensory cortical neurons,[93] there are relatively few which address the impact of specific transmitter manipulations upon SEPs. One of the most compelling demonstrated that SEPs of cats produced by forepaw stimulation were sensitive to minute quantities of topically applied GABA.[94] Under normal conditions, stimulation produced a forepaw SEP in primary somatosensory cortex of anesthetized cats which was characterized by a P1 (P11) and N1 (N20) wave. Application of 10 mg GABA completely abolished N1, suggesting an important role for this inhibitory transmitter in modulating N1 amplitude. Curiously, this effect of GABA could not be blocked by either picrotoxin or bicuculline.

C. Neurotoxicology

SEPs have been used occasionally, but not extensively, to detect and characterize neurotoxicity. It has been argued that toxicologists might use EPs for detection of diffuse CNS dysfunction as well as dysfunction specific to the sensory system under test.[5] The previously described studies which reported enhanced amplitude of SEP peaks in cases where damage was not in the primary somatosensory system support this point.[57] For screening purposes, SEPs offer two theoretical advantages over other sensory EPs. Transmission from the periphery to the cortex requires activity in such long tracts that extensive opportunity is provided (1) for toxicants to produce dysfunction and (2) if the dysfunction is diffuse, for it to be exaggerated or multiplied as successive long segments of the pathway are traversed. To date no data support these theoretical advantages.

Rebert[95] has made a case for inclusion of SEPs in a multisensory EP battery for detection and characterization of neurotoxicity. In these studies, rats with chronically implanted skull electrodes for recording SEPs were placed in a tubular restraining device and studied unanesthetized. Stimuli were delivered to the tip of the tail, presumably activating the ventral caudal nerve. However, to date, no publications have demonstrated that this preparation detects diffuse CNS dysfunction following exposure of adults to toxicants more effectively than EPs in other sensory systems or from simply recording the action potential from the caudal nerve.[96]

Several investigators have used SEPs to study the influence of perinatal exposure to potentially toxic substances upon the normal development of the somatosensory system. Salas and Schapior[37] administered either cortisol or thyroxin to rats on postnatal days 1, 2, and 3, and recorded EPs to somatosensory (sciatic), visual, and auditory stimuli on postnatal days 6, 9, 12, 15, 18, and 150. The recordings were made under anesthesia, with the skull exposed. A curious bipolar montage, with two surface electrodes separated by 2 to 3 mm, makes interpretation of the waveforms difficult. However, the authors reported that thyroxin-treated rats had an accelerated course of SEP development, while cortisol treated rats had a retarded course of development. The effects observed were even more prominent in the visual system than in the somatosensory system. The small numbers of rats and the apparent unavailability of a signal averager further hinders evaluation of this study, but the results are provocative since they suggest long-term modulation of sensory development by early hormonal processes.[97] Similar studies have indicated that malnutrition also retards the development of the rat SEP,[98] although effects upon secondary responses were even greater than on the primary response to sciatic stimulation.

Laurie and Boyes[38] recorded SEPs and VEPs in rats following neonatal exposure to diesel exhaust. While little consideration has been given by others to the potential influence of diesel exhaust on the nervous system, Laurie and Boyes[38] reported that SEPs recorded following tibial nerve stimulation were abnormal in the treated animals. Latencies of all peaks were prolonged on about postnatal day 14, and the recoverability of P2 amplitude in a paired stimulation paradigm was impaired on the same day. Changes similar to these were found in the visual system, where one peak exhibited a treatment induced increase in latency. In this case it is difficult to conclude that the somatosensory system was uniquely sensitive, but it may have been slightly more sensitive than the visual system.

It is well known that exposure to lead can slow conduction velocity in peripheral nerves.[99] It has also been reported that lead toxicity is detected by SEPs more readily than by conduction velocity.[100] The latter finding might reflect greater sensitivity of sensory fibers activated during SEP tests than mixed sensory and motor fibers activated during peripheral conduction tests, but the nature of the lead-induced change suggests that this is not the case. Seppalainen[100] reported 80% increase in the amplitude of the N1-P1 (N18-P22) peak evoked by median nerve stimulation and recorded from rolandic cortex of workers with occupational history of exposure to lead. This finding is illustrated in Figure 14. As noted previously, increased amplitudes are often associated with cortical damage distant from the recording site. Since only six subjects were involved in the high-level exposure group, caution is advised in

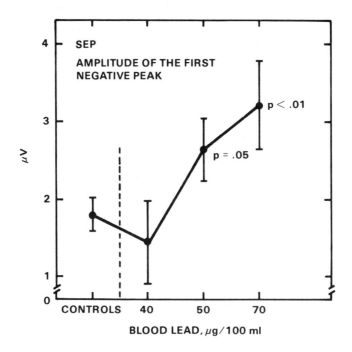

FIGURE 14.   Mean (± SEM) peak-to-peak amplitude of N1P1(N18-P22) of the SEP recorded from C4 among subjects with different maximal blood lead levels.[100]

generalizing from these data. Further, the absence of data comparing the effects of lead upon SEPs to the effects of lead on other sensory systems makes evaluation of the sensitivity of the method and the specificity of the effect difficult. When exposure to lead occurs during the perinatal period, rats have definite visual system dysfunction.[101]

SEPs appear to have been most useful to toxicologists when there were *a priori* reasons to suspect involvement of the somatosensory system. In such cases, recording SEPs can be used to (1) verify involvement of the system, (2) point to the locus of involvement within the system, and (3) trace in vivo the time course of involvement of different structures within the system. For example, Howell et al.[24] suspected involvement of the somatosensory system in rats treated with trimethyltin (TMT). TMT-treated Long-Evans hooded rats engaged in a pattern of self-mutilation of the tail which suggested deafferentation. A hot plate test for behavioral reactivity to thermal pain also suggested somatosensory dysfunction, since TMT-treated rats took longer than controls to exhibit signs of discomfort. Evaluation of threshold and conduction velocity in the dorsal caudal tail nerve revealed no peripheral dysfunction, but SEPs recorded from the skull following tail nerve stimulation had longer latencies and smaller amplitudes in TMT-treated rats than in controls. The SEP technique thereby verified the existence of dysfunction in the somatosensory system, and repeated recordings demonstrated the progressive nature of dysfunction. While the suggestion was made that the findings indicated central and not peripheral dysfunction, the absence of alterations in nerve conduction velocity may have reflected a blurring of effect due to the mix of sensory and motor fibers involved in the conduction velocity measurement.

Leitch and Hallenbeck[102] used SEPs to monitor the dysfunction produced by spinal cord decompression sickness in dogs. SEP amplitude changes appeared to correlate with changes in cerebral blood flow, although the small number of dogs studied (n = 7) makes quantitative descriptions difficult.

Hexacarbons produce a neuropathy often described as central-peripheral distal axonopathy.[103] In cases of hexacarbon toxicity, both ends of the first-order neuron undergo toxic changes, such that pathology may be observed in the periphery and in the rostral extent of the dorsal columns. Since slowing of peripheral nerve conduction appears to precede clinical signs in *n*-hexane neurotoxicity,[104] recording SEPs from *n*-hexane-exposed subjects should provide an even more sensitive indicator of neurotoxicity, requiring as it does conduction along both peripheral and central segments of the first order neuron.

Mutti et al.[105] recorded SEPs following median nerve stimulation in shoe factory workers with known occupational exposure (2 to 8 years) to hexane, cyclohexane, methyl-ethyl ketone, and ethyl acetate. Recordings were made between 3 and 6 months after removal from exposure, so that all effects observed were considered chronic, and results were compared to an age-matched population of shoe factory workers with no known history of exposure to these solvents. As expected, the exposed workers had significantly decreased conduction velocities in peripheral nerves. However, there was only a slight increase in latency of peak N1 (N20) recorded from the scalp. The effect of exposure upon early components of the SEP appeared to be a disruption of the "W" response.[45] Much more impressive than the disrupted "W" response was the flattening of the later peaks (those occurring after 40 msec) in exposed subjects. The surprising feature of this study was the more robust detection of exposure by the peripheral nerve conduction velocity than by the SEP. The relative failure of the SEP in this study might reflect greater variability of measures of cerebral compared to peripheral activity, or might in some way reflect the late postexposure nature of the recordings. However, the latter would seem, on the surface, to favor SEPs over peripheral nerve recordings.

In contrast to the Mutti et al.[105] study, Thomas et al.,[106] who exposed baboons to 2,5-hexanedione, found increased SEP latencies and decreased peripheral nerve conduction velocities. Both measures were effective in detecting toxicity. These studies were done during the period of acute toxicity and under anesthesia. An interesting comparison was made between the effects of 2,5-hexanedione and the effects of clioquinol. Clioquinol, a halogenated hydroxyquinoline used as an antimicrobial agent, produces damage in the centrally directed axons of dorsal root ganglion neurons, while sparing the peripherally directed axons.[106] As expected, clioquinol produced little effect upon peripheral nerve conduction velocities. Peak P1 SEP latencies were significantly increased following stimulation of either the lower limb or the upper limb, but the magnitude of delay was substantially less than was observed in the 2,5-hexanedione-treated baboons. Unfortunately, SEP amplitudes were not reported in this study, perhaps due to difficulties the authors indicated maintaining consistent levels of anesthesia. Both groups of treated animals exhibited similar clinical signs (lethargy, ataxia, paraparesis, hypotonia, and piloerection), and neuropathological findings were consistent with expectations based upon previous studies. In this study, then, SEPs added little to the conduction velocity data in the 2,5-hexanedione case. In the case of clioquinol, the combined use of peripheral nerve conduction and SEP studies allowed an accurate assessment of the locus of damage.

Acrylamide is another neurotoxic substance which produces a central-peripheral axonopathy. Boyes et al.[108] recorded SEPs produced by tibial nerve stimulation from rats exposed to acrylamide. The findings were surprising, because latency to N1, the second cortical peak in rats, was affected following fewer exposures than was latency to P1, the first cortical peak. Since any peripheral damage should have been reflected in a P1 latency shift, these data suggest that the central nervous system may be affected by acrylamide neurotoxicity more rapidly than the peripheral nervous system. Peaks beyond N1 were evidently unaffected. In a subsequent study using higher concentrations of acrylamide, Boyes and Cooper[109] recorded far-field SEPs from rats after 4, 8, and 16 days of exposure to 400 ppm acrylamide in drinking water. No changes were evident until the 16th day, at which point the cumulative dose was about 600 mg/kg. On day 16 latencies of peaks II, III, and P1 were significantly increased, while latency of peak I was not. Similarly, amplitude of peaks II, III, and P1

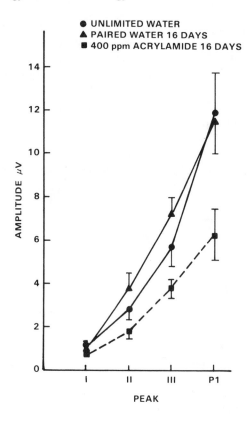

FIGURE 15.   Mean (± SEM) far-field SEP amplitudes
recorded from rats given either unlimited access to water,
paired water, or 400 ppm and acrylamide in water daily
for 16 days.[109]

were significantly decreased. The amplitude data are depicted in Figure 15. These findings
also support the interpretation that central damage occurs prior to peripheral damage, although
it should be noted that the stimulation site was at the ankle, above the nerve terminals,
which should show the earliest peripheral damage. Therefore, the study was biased in favor
of finding a CNS change first. In contrast to the findings of Perbellini et al.[104] with *n*-hexane,
Boyes and Cooper[109] observed clinical signs of toxicity prior to electrophysiological signs
of toxicity.

More recently, Arezzo et al.[110] performed a similar experiment in monkeys *(Macaca
fascicularis)*, injecting 10 mg/kg acrylamide subcutaneously 6 days/week. One monkey each
was injected for 5, 15, 16, 50, and 83 days, and recordings were made once or twice a
week. In this study, electrophysiological data recorded from the scalp were compared to (1)
clinical signs of toxicity, (2) peripheral nerve conduction velocities, (3) evoked potentials
recorded over the spinal cord, and (4) neuropathological findings. The results indicated
clearly that conduction velocity and amplitude changes in the terminal and preterminal axons
of the fasciculus gracilis preceded more peripherally occurring changes, and that these
changes correlated well with the onset of neuropathological changes. The authors did not
indicate whether more rostrally generated peaks were affected even earlier. In contrast to
Boyes and Cooper,[109] electrophysiological changes preceded clinical signs of toxicity.

In conclusion, SEPs and FFSEPs have been used only occasionally in studies of neurotoxicity. When dysfunction is diffuse, affecting more than one system, SEPs do not appear
to have properties which recommend them more highly than evoked potential tests of other
sensory systems. So few studies have employed SEPs in this context that one must reserve

final judgment on this issue. However, when specific toxicity to the somatosensory system is suspected, SEPs may be useful in verifying toxicity and in pointing to the most sensitive links in the somatosensory chain. There is still disagreement regarding whether SEP changes may be observed prior to clinical signs of toxicity, but it seems reasonable to suppose that the resolution of this disagreement will depend upon the rigor of the respective clinical and electrophysiological examinations, the nature of the toxicant, the species, and the number of subjects tested. It is not clear that resolution of the relative sensitivity of behavioral, physiological, or other end-points has practical importance. It seems evident that all will continue to be useful, for all but the most rudimentary screening purposes, in the foreseeable future.

V. PERFORMING SEP STUDIES

To perform an adequate SEP study, many decisions must be made, including selection and preparation of the subjects, and details of the stimulation and recording situation. In most cases, the choices made will depend upon the nature of the questions posed by the investigator, and the preceding sections should be useful in helping the reader to make informed decisions. In the following sections, a few of the choice points will be identified.

A. Experimental Design
It is the nature of EP experiments in general that a multitude of end-points are almost as easily acquired as a single end-point. Thus, it is nearly as simple to measure all detectable peak amplitudes and latencies of a waveform as it is to measure only one. While this approach is essential for exploring one's data and designing future studies, it is rarely appreciated that including all of these variables in formal statistical analyses virtually assures (by chance) finding a "significant" effect. Detailed strategies for successfully dealing with this problem are outlined by Muller et al.[111] An important take-home message is that every effort should be made to (1) maximize the number of subjects tested, (2) minimize the number of dependent variables measured, and (3) minimize the number of independent variables manipulated. All of these measures will increase the power of statistical tests performed.

Not all studies are performed with the intent to make statements regarding the statistical probability of a particular effect. Many studies are intentionally qualitative, deal with only a few subjects, and may be best described as "demonstrations". For example, only a demonstration study is required to show that a particular waveform reverses polarity as the cortex is traversed. Demonstration-type studies play a valuable role, but they should never be confused with statistically rigorous studies. Unfortunately, the literature is replete with such confusion because investigators who perform demonstration studies tend to pepper them with non-Bonferroni-corrected "t" tests, lending a superficial aura of statistical respectability. Because toxicological studies with relevance to public health may be used in court cases, it is necessary that they be particularly rigorous, and caution is therefore recommended.

B. Selecting the Subject
As described previously, species, age, size, and gender are all important determinants of SEP waveforms. While the decisions will depend upon the nature of the questions posed, it makes sense to think in terms of rodents for statistically controlled studies, because they are sufficiently economical to allow adequate sample sizes, and to think in terms of nonhuman primates for demonstration studies, because they are most like humans. Peculiarities of toxicant metabolism may conflict with the need to choose a cost-effective species although in most cases information on metabolism is not available.

C. Preparing the Subject
Once the subjects have been selected, the nature of the subject preparation must be

determined. Will the electrodes be chronic, or will they be placed at the time of recording? The former guarantees identical placement when multiple recordings are to be made, but also requires surgery with the attendent risks of infection. Will the subject be tested while anesthetized? Use of anesthesia, by relieving concerns about pain and movement artifacts, allows incorporation of higher stimulus intensities, thereby activating slower-conducting axons. On the other hand, both anesthesia and intense stimulation are likely to produce results with questionable generality to the normal functioning organism. In some cases such a generality may be more important than others. In toxicological studies one runs the risk of using an anesthetic which interacts with the toxicant under study to produce a result which would not be observed in an unanesthesized subject.

Whether the subject is anesthetized or unanesthetized, care must be taken to ensure that temperature is controlled. Rectal temperature is not a good predictor of skin or nerve temperature, but when rectal temperature is not changing, it is a fairly good predictor of brain temperature. SEP studies must be concerned with both brain and nerve temperature, although neither have been given sufficient attention in the literature.

D. Decisions about Stimulating and Recording

The decisions required for most EP studies also apply here. One must decide upon a location for the active recording electrodes, a decision which may rest upon studies demonstrating the topographical distribution of the waveform on the surface of the brain. The topographical distribution of the waveform in turn depends upon the location of the stimulating electrode. Perhaps equally important is location of the reference electrode. As indicated above, a truly indifferent electrode is particularly difficult to find in FFSEP studies.

The characteristics of the recording amplifier (gain, coupling, and bandpass) depend upon the waveform as well. Studies of far-field responses require amplifiers with greater gain and a higher frequency response than do studies which focus upon later responses. Recommendations for bandpass settings are available from the literature, but care must be taken to ensure that the rolloff of the filters is understood before recommendation of others are applied routinely.[112,113] The epoch length and the number of trials to average are often matters of personal preference, but the A/D conversion rate should exceed the highest frequency of the signal to be recognized by at least a factor of two.

Location of the stimulating electrodes, type of stimulating electrode, type of stimulus (mechanical vs. electrical), stimulus intensity, and stimulus rate all depend upon the specific questions the investigator intends to answer. In performing electrical stimulation studies, one does well to keep in mind some basic relationships between the stimulus properties and the properties of the tissue the stimulus is supposed to activate.[114]

Traditionally, analyses of SEPs have been performed upon peak latencies, onset latencies, peak to peak amplitudes, and/or baseline to peak amplitudes. Interpeak latencies have been used to describe central conduction time, and an RMS measure of amplitude may be appropriate for a screening-type exam. Other possibilities include spectral analysis of the waveform, and variability analysis.[115] However, it is worth worrying about data which are so highly derived that all intuitive explanatory value is lost.

ACKNOWLEDGMENTS

The careful typing of the text by Judy Smith is greatly appreciated. Appreciation is also extended to Will Boyes for thoughtful discussions and for critical comments.

REFERENCES

1. **Darian-Smith, I.,** Thermal sensibility, in *Handbook of Physiology,* Section I, Vol III, Part 2, Darian-Smith, I., Ed., American Physiological Society, Bethesda, Md., 1984, 879.
2. **Mountcastle, V. B.,** Mechanoreceptive sensibility, in *Handbook of Physiology,* Section I, Vol. III, Part 2, Darian-Smith, I., Ed., American Physiological Society, Bethesda, Md., 1984, 789.
3. **Perl, E. R.,** Pain and nociception, in *Handbook of Physiology,* Section I, Vol. III, Part 2, Darian-Smith, I., Ed., American Physiological Society, Bethesda, Md., 1984, 915.
4. **Fleming, D. E., Shearer, D. E., and Creel, D. J.,** Effect of pharmacologically-induced arousal on the evoked potential in the unanesthetized rat, *Pharmacol. Biochem. Behav.,* 2, 187, 1974.
5. **Dyer, R. S.,** Neurophysiological measures following exposure to toxic substances, in *Behavioral Toxicology,* Annual, Z., Ed., Johns Hopkins, Baltimore, 1985.
6. **Hume, A. L. and Cant, B. R.,** Conduction time in central somatosensory pathways in man, *Electroencephalog. Clin. Neurophysiol.,* 45, 361, 1978.
7. **Arezzo, J. C. Vaughan, H. G., and Legatt, A. D.,** Topography and intracranial sources of somatosensory evoked potentials in the monkey. II. Cortical components, *Electroencephalog. Clin. Neurophysiol.,* 51, 1, 1981.
8. **Desmedt, J. E., Huy, N. T., and Bourguet, M.,** The cognitive P40, N60 and P100 components of somatosensory evoked potentials and the earliest electrical signs of sensory processing in man, *Electroencephalog. Clin. Neurophysiol.,* 56, 272, 1983.
9. **Desmedt, J. E. and Cheron, G.,** Somatosensory evoked potentials in man: subcortical and cortical components and their neural basis, *Ann. N.Y. Acad. Sci.,* 388, 388, 1982.
10. **Dong, W. K. and Chudler, E. H.,** Origins of tooth pulp-evoked farfield and early near-field potentials in the cat, *J. Neurophysiol.,* 51, 859, 1984.
11. **Kimura, J., Mitsudome, A., Yamada, T., and Dickens, Q. S.,** Stationary peaks from a moving source in far-field recording, *Electroencephalog. Clin. Neurophysiol.,* 58, 351, 1984.
12. **Allison, T. and Hume, A. L.,** A comparative analysis of short-latency somatosensory evoked potentials in man, monkey, cat and rat, *Exp. Neurol.,* 72, 592, 1981.
13. **Allison, T., Wood, C. C., McCarthy, G., Hume, A. L., and Goff, W. R.,** Short-latency somatosensory evoked potentials in man, monkey, cat and rat: comparative latency analysis, in *Clinical Applications of Evoked Potentials in Neurology,* Courjon, J., Mauguiere, F., and Revol, M., Eds., Raven Press, New York, 1982, 303.
14. **Wiederholt, W. C. and Iragui-Madoz, V. J.,** Far-field somatosensory potentials in the rat, *Electroencephalog. Clin. Neurophysiol.,* 42, 456, 1977.
15. **Arezzo, J., Legatt, A. D., and Vaughan, H. G.,** Topography and intracranial sources of somatosensory evoked potentials in the monkey. I. Early components, *Electroencephalog. Clin. Neurophysiol.,* 46, 155, 1979.
16. **Hashimoto, I.,** Somatosensory evoked potentials from the human brain-stem: origins of short latency potentials, *Electroencephalog. Clin. Neurophysiol.,* 57, 221, 1984.
17. **Suzuki, I. and Mayanagi, Y.,** Intracranial recording of short latency somatosensory evoked potentials in man: identification of origin of each component, *Electroencephalog. Clin. Neurophysiol.,* 59, 286, 1984.
18. **Jewett, D. L., Romano, M. N., and Williston, J. S.,** Human auditory evoked potentials: possible brainstem components detected on the scalp, *Science,* 167, 1516, 1970.
19. **Ganes, T.,** A study of peripheral, cervical and cortical evoked potentials and afferent conduction times in the somatosensory pathway, *Electroencephalog. Clin. Neurophysiol,* 49, 446, 1980.
20. **Rossini, P. M. and Treviso, M.,** Central conduction velocity (lumbar-vertex) in man calculated by means of a new method. Studies on variability, the effects of sex, age and different equipments, *Eur. Neurol.,* 22, 173, 1983.
21. **Welker, W. I. and Seidenstein, S.,** Somatic sensory representation in the cerebral cortex of the racoon (Procyon lotor), *J. Comp. Neurol.,* 111, 469, 1959.
22. **Welker, C.,** Microelectrode delineation of fine grain somatotopic organization of SmI cerebral neocortex in albino rat, *Brain Res.,* 26, 259, 1971.
23. **Weinberg, R., Barbaresi, P., Cheema, S., Spreafico, R., and Rustioni, A.,** SI and SII projections from somatosensory thalamus of rats, *Neurosci. Abstr.,* 10, 945, 1984.
24. **Howell, W. E., Walsh, T. J., and Dyer, R. S.,** Trimethyltin produces somatosensory dysfunction, *Neurobehav. Toxicol. Teratol.,* 4, 196, 1982.
25. **Rebert, C. S. and Sorenson, S. S.,** Concentration-related effects of hexane on evoked responses from brain and peripheral nerve of the rat, *Neurobehav. Toxicol. Teratol.,* 5, 69, 1983.
26. **Chapin, J. K. and Lin, C.-S.,** Mapping the body representation in the SI cortex of anesthetized and awake rats, *J. Comp. Neurol.,* 229, 199, 1984.
27. **Hall, R. D. and Lindholm, E. P.,** Organization of motor and somatosensory neocortex in the albino rat, *Brain Res.,* 66, 23, 1974.

28. **Miyoshi, T. and Goto, I.,** Serial in vivo determinations of nerve conduction velocity in rat tails. Physiological and pathological changes, *Electroencephalog. Clin. Neurophysiol.,* 35, 125, 1973.

29. **Glatt, A. F., Talaat, H. N., and Koella, W. P.,** Testing of peripheral nerve function in chronic experiments in rats, *Pharmacol. Ther.,* 5, 539, 1979.

30. **Isseroff, R. G., Sarne, Y., Carmon, A., and Isseroff, A.,** Cortical potentials evoked by innocuous tactile and noxious thermal stimulation in the rat: differences in localization and latency, *Behav. Neurol. Biol.,* 35, 294, 1982.

31. **Purpura, D. P., Shofer, R. J., Housepian, E. M., and Noback, C. R.,** Comparative ontogenesis of structure-function relations in cerebral and cerebellar cortex, *Prog. Brain Res.,* 4, 187, 1964.

32. **Molliver, M. E.,** An ontogenic study of evoked somesthetic cortical responses in the sheep, *Dev. Neurol.,* 26, 78, 1967.

33. **Marty, R.,** Développment post-natal des réponse sensorielles du cortex cérébral chez le chat et le lapin, *Arch. Anat. Micr. Morph. Exp.,* 51, 129, 1962.

34. **Desmedt, J. E.,** Somatosensory cerebral evoked potentials in man, in *Handbook of EEG and Clinical Neurophysiology,* Vol. 9, Remond, A., Ed., Elsevier, Amsterdam, 1971, 55.

35. **Desmedt, J. E., Brunko, E., and Debecker, J.,** Maturation of the somatosensory evoked potentials in normal infants and children, with special reference to the early N1 component, *Electroencephalog. Clin. Neurophysiol.,* 40, 43, 1976.

36. **Mares, P. and Faladova, L.,** Development of cortical somatosensory evoked potentials in rats, *Acta Biol. Med. Germ.,* 34, 1013, 1975.

37. **Salas, M. and Schapiro, S.,** Hormonal influences upon the maturation of the rat brain's responsiveness to sensory stimuli, *Physiol. Behav.,* 5, 1970.

38. **Laurie, R. D. and Boyes, W. K.,** Neurophysiological alterations due to diesel exhaust exposure during the neonatal life of the rat, *Environ. Int.,* 5, 363, 1981.

39. **Desmedt, J. E. and Cheron, G.,** Somatosensory evoked potentials to finger stimulation in healthy octogenarians and in young adults: wave forms, scalp topography and transit times of parietal and frontal components, *Electroencephalog. Clin. Neurophysiol.,* 50, 404, 1980.

40. **Allison, T., Hume, A. L., Wood, C. C., and Goff, W. R.,** Developmental and aging changes in somatosensory, auditory and visual evoked potentials, *Electroencephalog. Clin. Neurophysiol.,* 58, 14,

41. **Simpson, D. M. and Erwin, C. W.,** Evoked potential latency change with age suggests differential aging of primary somatosensory cortex, *Neurobiol. Aging,* 4, 59, 1983.

42. **Dyer, R. S. and Swartzwelder, H. S.,** Sex and strain differencies in the visual evoked potentials of albino and hooded rats, *Pharmacol. Biochem. Behav.,* 9, 301, 1978.

43. **Ikuta, T. and Furuta, N.,** Sex differences in the human group mean SEP, *Electroencephalog. Clin. Neurophysiol.,* 54, 449, 1982.

44. **Soininen, K. and Jarvilehto, T.,** Somatosensory evoked potentials associated with tactile stimulation at detection thresholds in man, *Electroencephalog. Clin. Neurophysiol.,* 56, 494, 1983.

45. **Giblin, D. R.,** Scalp-recorded somatosensory evoked potentials, in *Electrodiagnosis in Clinical Neurology,* Aminoff, M. J., Ed., Churchill Livingstone, New York, 1980, 414.

46. **Young, R. F. and King, R. B.,** Fibre spectrum of the trigeminal root of the baboon by electron microscopy, *J. Neurosurg.,* 38, 65, 1973.

47. **Harkins, S. W. and Chapma, C. R.,** Cerebral evoked potentials to noxious dental stimulation: relationship to subjective pain report, *Psychophysiology,* 15, 248, 1978.

48. **Rohdewald, P., Derendorf, H., Drehesen, G., Elger, C. E., and Knoll, O.,** Changes in cortical evoked potentials as correlates of the efficacy of weak analgesics, *Pain,* 12, 329, 1982.

49. **Crucco, G., Fornarelli, M., Inghilleri, M., and Manf, M.,** The limits of tooth pulp evoked potentials for pain quantitation, *Physiol. Behav.,* 31, 339, 1983.

50. **Anziska, B. and Cracco, R. Q.,** Short latency somatosensory evoked potentials: studies in patients with focal neurological disease, *Neurology,* 49, 227, 1980.

51. **Schiff, J. A., Cracco, R. Q., Rossini, P. M., and Cracco, J. B.,** Spine and spinal somatosensory evoked potentials in normal subjects and patients with spinal cord disease: evaluation of afferent transmission, *Electroencephalog. Clin. Neurophysiol.,* 59, 374, 1984.

52. **Desmedt, J. E. and Noel, P.,** Average cerebral evoked potentials in the evaluation of lesions of the sensory nerves and of central somatosensory pathways, in *New Developments in Electromyography and Clinical Neurophysiology,* Vol. 2, Desmedt, J. E., Ed., Karger, Basal, 1973, 352.

53. **Powers, S. K., Bolger, C. A., and Edwards, M. S. B.,** Spinal cord pathways mediating somatosensory evoked potentials, *J. Neurosurg.,* 57, 472, 1982.

54. **Yamada, T., Kimura, J., Wilkinson, J. T., and Kayamori, R.,** Short- and long-latency median somatosensory evoked potentials. Findings in patients with localized neurological lesions, *Arch. Neurol.,* 40, 215, 1983.

55. **Stohr, M., Dichgans, J., Voigt, K., and Buettner, U. W.,** The significance of somatosensory evoked potentials for localization of unilateral lesions within the cerebral hemispheres, *J. Neurol. Sci.,* 61, 49, 1983.
56. **Mauguiere, F., Desmedt, J. E., and Courjon, J.,** Astereognosis and dissociated loss of frontal or parietal components of somatosensory evoked potentials in hemispheric lesions, *Brain,* 106, 271, 1983.
57. **Obeso, J. A., Marti-Masso, J. F., and Carrera, N.,** Somatosensory evoked potentials: abnormalities with focal brain lesions remote from the primary sensorimotor area, *Electroencephalog. Clin. Neurophysiol.,* 49, 59, 1980.
58. **Bigum, H. B., Dustman, R. E., and Beck, E. C.,** Visual and somatosensory evoked responses from mongoloid and normal children, *Electroencephalog. Clin. Neurophysiol.,* 28, 576, 1970.
59. **Watson, R. T., Miller, B. D., and Heilman, K. M.,** Evoked potentials in neglect, *Arch. Neurol.,* 34, 24, 1977.
60. **Majkowski, J. and Kwast, O.,** Changes in somatosensory evoked potentials during kindling: analogy to learning modifications, *Epilepsia,* 22, 267, 1981.
61. **Shibasaki, H., Yamashita, Y., and Kuroiwa, Y.,** Electroencephalographic studies of myoclonus, *Brain,* 101, 447, 1978.
62. **Rothwell, J. C., Obeso, J. A., and Marsden, C. D.,** On the significance of giant somatosensory evoked potentials in cortical myoclonus, *J. Neurol. Neurosurg. Psychiatr.,* 47, 33, 1984.
63. **Takahashi, H. and Straschill, M.,** The effects of focal epileptic activity on the somatosensory evoked potentials in the rat, *Arch. Psychiatr. Nervenkr.,* 231, 81, 1981.
64. **Josiassen, R. C., Shagass, C., Mancall, E. L., and Roemer, R. A.,** Somatosensory evoked potentials in Huntington's Disease, *Electroencephalog. Clin. Neurophysiol.,* 54, 483, 1982.
65. **Noth, J., Engle, L., Friedemann, H.-H., and Lange, H. W.,** Evoked potentials in patients with Huntington's Disease and their offspring. I. Somatosensory evoked potentials, *Electroencephalog. Clin. Neurophysiol.,* 59, 134, 1984.
66. **Aminoff, M. J., Davis, S. L., and Panitch, H. S.,** Serial evoked potential studies in patients with definite multiple sclerosis, clinical relevance, *Arch. Neurol.,* 41, 1197, 1984.
67. **Walsh, J. C., Garrick, R., Cameron, J., and Mcleod, J. G.,** Evoked potentials in clinically definite multiple sclerosis: a two year follow-up study, *J. Neurol. Neurosurg. Psychiatr.,* 45, 494, 1982.
68. **Purvis, S. J., Low, M. D., Galloway, J., and Reeves, B.,** A comparison of visual, brainstem auditory, and somatosensory evoked potentials in multiple sclerosis, *Can. J. Neurol. Sci.,* 8, 15, 1981.
69. **Phillips, K. R., Potvin, A. R., Syndulko, K., Cohen, S. N., Tourtellotte, W. W., and Potvin, J. H.,** Multimodality evoked potentials and neurophysiological tests in multiple sclerosis. Effects of hyperthermia on test results, *Arch. Neurol.,* 40, 159, 1983.
70. **Kazis, A., Vlaikidis, N., Xafenias, D., Papanastasiou, J., and Pappa, P.,** Fever and evoked potentials in multiple sclerosis, *J. Neurol.,* 227, 1, 1982.
71. **Matthews, W. B., Read, D. J., and Pountney, E.,** Effect of raising body temperature on visual and somatosensory evoked potentials in patients with multiple sclerosis, *J. Neurol. Neurosurg. Psychiatr.,* 42, 250, 1979.
72. **Cosi, V., Poloni, M., Mazzini, L., and Callieco, R.,** Somatosensory evoked potentials in amyotrophic lateral sclerosis, *J. Neurol. Neurosurg. Psychiatr.,* 47, 857, 1984.
73. **Abbruzzese, G., Reni, L., Copcito, L., Ratto, S., Abbruzzese, M., and Favale, E.,** Short-latency somatosensory evoked potentials in degenerative and vascular dementia, *J. Neurol. Neurosurg. Psychiatr.,* 47, 1034, 1984.
74. **Rumpl, E., Prugger, M., Gerstenbrand, F., Hackl, J. M., and Pallua, A.,** Central somatosensory conduction time and short latency somatosensory evoked potentials in post-traumatic coma, *Electroencephalog. Clin. Neurophysiol.,* 56, 583, 1983.
75. **de la Torre, J. C.,** Evaluation of brain death using somatosensory evoked potentials, *Biol. Psychiatr.,* 16, 931, 1981.
76. **de la Torre, J. C., Trimble, J. L., Beard, R. T., Hanlon, K., and Surgeon, J. W.,** Somatosensory evoked potentials for the prognosis of coma in humans, *Exp. Neurol.,* 60, 304, 1978.
77. **Hume, A. L., Cant, B. R., and Shaw, N. A.,** Central somatosensory conduction time in comatose patients, *Ann. Neurol.,* 5, 379, 1979.
78. **Goff, W. R., Shaywitz, B. A., Goff, G. D., Reisenauer, M. A., Kasiorkowsi, J. G., Venes, J. L., and Rothstein, P. T.,** Somatic evoked potential evaluation of cerebral status in Reye syndrome, *Electroencephalog. Clin. Neurophysiol.,* 55, 388, 1983.
79. **Lesser, R. P., Lueders, H., Hahn, J., and Klem, G.,** Early somatosensory potentials evoked by median nerve stimulation: intraoperative monitoring, *Neurology,* 31, 1519, 1981.
80. **Lueders, H., Lesser, R., Gurd, A., and Klem, G.,** Recovery functions of spinal cord and subcortical somatosensory evoked potentials to posterior tibial nerve stimulation: intrasurgical recordings, *Brain Res.,* 309, 27, 1984.

81. **Macon, J. B. and Poletti, C. E.,** Conducted somatosensory evoked potentials during spinal surgery. I. Control conduction velocity measurements, *J. Neurosurg.,* 57, 349, 1982.
82. **Markand, O. N., Dilley, R. S., Moorthy, S. S., and Warren, C.,** Monitoring of somatosensory evoked responses during carotid endartectomy, *Arch. Neurol.,* 41, 375, 1984.
83. **Sutton, L. N., Frewen, T., Marsh, R., Jaggi, J., and Bruce, D. A.,** The effects of deep barbiturate coma on multimodality evoked potentials, *J. Neurosurg.,* 57, 178, 1982.
84. **Clark, D. L., Hosick, C. E., and Rosner, B. S.,** Neurophysiological effects of different anesthetics in unconscious man, *J. Appl. Physiol.,* 31, 884, 1971.
85. **Pathak, K. S., Brown, R. H., Cascorbi, H. F., and Nash, C. L., Jr.,** Effects of fentanyl and morphine on interoperative somatosensory cortical-evoked potentials, *Anesth. Analg.,* 62, 833, 1984.
86. **Ganes, T. and Lundar, T.,** The effect of thiopentone on somatosensory evoked responses and EEGs in comatose patients, *J. Neurol. Neurosurg. Psychiatry,* 46, 509, 1983.
87. **Angel, A., Gratton, D. A., Halsey, M. J., and Wardley-Smith, B.,** Pressure reversal of the effect of urethane on the evoked somatosensory cortical response in the rat, *Br. J. Pharmacol.,* 70, 241, 1980.
88. **Dyer, R. S. and Boyes, W. K.,** Hypothermia and anesthesia differentially affect the flash evoked potentials of hooded rats, *Brain Res. Bull.,* 10, 825, 1983.
89. **Hetzler, B. E. and Dyer, R. S.,** Contribution of hypothermia to effects of chloral hydrate on flash evoked potentials of hooded rats, *Pharmacol. Biochem. Behav.,* 21, 599, 1984.
90. **Stejskal, L., Travnicek, V., Sourek, K., and Kredba, J.,** Somatosensory evoked potentials in deep hypothermia, *Appl. Neurophysiol.,* 43, 1, 1980.
91. **Britt, R. H., Lyons, B. E., Ryan, T., Saxer, E., Obana, W., and Rossi, G.,** Effect of whole-body hyperthermia on auditory brainstem and somatosensory and visual evoked potentials, in *Thermal Physiology,* Hales, J. R. S., Ed., Raven Press, New York 1984, 519.
92. **Budnick, B., McKeown, K. L., and Wiederholt, W. C.,** Hypothermia-induced changes in rat short latency somatosensory evoked potentials, *Electroencephalog. Clin. Neurophysiol.,* 51, 19, 1981.
93. **Dykes, R. W., Landry, P., Metherate, R., and Hicks, T. P.,** Functional role of GABA in cat primary somatosensory cortex: shaping receptive fields or cortical neurons, *J. Neurophysiol.,* 52, 1066, 1984.
94. **Brailowsky, S. and Knight, R. T.,** Inhibitory modulation of cat somatosensory cortex: a pharmacological study, *Brain Res.,* 322, 310, 1984.
95. **Rebert, C. S.,** Multisensory evoked potentials in experimental and applied neurotoxicology, *Neurobehav. Toxicol. Teratol.,* 5, 659, 1983.
96. **Rebert, C. S., Pryor, G. T., and Frick, M. S.,** Effects of vincristine, maytansine and cis-platinum on behavioral and electrophysiological indicies of neurotoxicity in the rat, *J. Appl. Toxicol.,* 4, 330, 1984.
97. **Salas, M., Diaz, S., and Cintra, L.,** Electrocortical effects of early postnatal thyroxine administration in the rat, *Physiol. Behav.,* 17, 239, 1976.
98. **Salas, M. and Cintra, L.,** Nutritional influences upon somatosensory evoked responses during development in the rat, *Physiol. Behav.,* 10, 1019, 1973.
99. **Singer, R., Valcuikas, J. A., and Lilis, R.,** Lead exposure and nerve conduction velocity: the differential time course of sensory and motor nerve effects, *Neurotoxicology,* 4(1), 193, 1983.
100. **Seppalainen, A. M.,** Diagnostic utility of neuroelectric measures in environmental and occupational medicine, in *Multidisciplinary Perspectives in Event-Related Brain Potential Research,* Otto, D. A., Ed., U.S. Environmental Protection Agency, Research Triangle Park, N.C., 1978, 448.
101. **Fox, D. A., Lewkowski, J. P., and Cooper, G. P.,** Acute and chronic effects of neonatal lead exposure on development of the visual evoked response in rats, *Toxicol. Appl. Pharmacol.,* 40, 449, 1977.
102. **Leitch, D. R. and Hallenbeck, J. M.,** Somatosensory evoked potentials and neuraxial blood flow in central nervous system decompression sickness, *Brain Res.,* 311, 307, 1984.
103. **Spencer, P. S. and Schaumburg, H. H.,** Classification of neurotoxic disease: a morphological approach, in *Experimental and Clinical Neurotoxicology,* Spencer, P. S. and Schaumburg, H. H., Eds., Williams & Wilkins, Baltimore, 1980, 92.
104. **Perbellini, L., de Grandis, D., Semenzato, F., Rizzuto, N., and Simonati, A.,** An experimental study of the neurotoxicity of *n*-hexane metabolites: hexanol-1 and hexanol-2, *Toxicol. Appl. Pharmacol.,* 46, 421, 1978.
105. **Mutti, A., Ferri, F., Lommi, G., Lotta, S., Lucertini, S., and Franchini, I.,** *n*-Hexane-induced changes in nerve conduction velocities and somatosensory evoked potentials, *Arch. Occup. Environ. Health,* 51, 45, 1982.
106. **Thomas, P. K., Bradley, D. J., Bradley, W. A., Degen, P. H., Krinke, G., Muddle, J., Schaumburg, H. H., Skelton-Stroud, P. N., Thomann, P., and Tzebelikos, E.,** Correlated nerve conduction, somatosensory evoked potential and neuropathological studies in clioquinol and 2.5-hexanedione neurotoxicity in the baboon, *J. Neurol. Sci.,* 64, 277, 1984.
107. **Thomas, P. K.,** Selective vulnerability of the centrifugal and centripetal axons of primary sensory neurons, *Muscle Nerve,* 5, 5117, 1982.

108. **Boyes, W. K., Laurie, R. D., and Cooper, G. P.,** Acrylamide toxicity: effects on cortical evoked potentials and locomotor activities in rats, *Neurosci. Abstr.,* 6, 727, 1980.

109. **Boyes, W. K. and Cooper, G. P.,** Acrylamide neurotoxicity: effects on far-field somatosensory evoked potentials in rats, *Neurobehav. Toxicol. Teratol.,* 3, 487, 1981.

110. **Arezzo, J. C., Schaumburg, H. H., and Spencer, P. S.,** Structure and function of the somatosensory system: a neurotoxicological perspective, *Environ. Health Perspect.,* 44, 23, 1982.

111. **Muller, K. E., Barton, C. N., and Benignus, V. A.,** Recommendations for appropriate statistical practice in toxicologic experiments, *Neurotoxicology,* 5, 113, 1984.

112. **Desmedt, J. E., Brunko, E., Debecker, J., and Carmeliet, J.,** The system bandpass required to avoid distortion of early components when averaging somatosensory evoked potentials, *Electroencephalog. Clin. Neurophysiol.,* 37, 407, 1974.

113. **Maccabee, P. J., Pinkhasov, E. I., and Cracco, R. Q.,** Short latency somatosensory evoked potentials to median nerve stimulation: effect of low frequency filter, *Electroencephalog. Clin. Neurophysiol.,* 55, 34, 1983.

114. **Ranck, J. B., Jr.,** Which elements are excited in electrical stimulation of mammalian central nervous system: a review, *Brain Res.,* 98, 417, 1975.

115. **Wong, P. K. H., Lombroso, C. T., and Matsumiya, Y.,** Somatosensory evoked potentials: variability analysis in unilateral hemispheric disease, *Electroencephalog. Clin. Neurophysiol.,* 54, 266, 1982.

116. **Dyer, R. S.,** Unpublished.

Chapter 6

SPINAL CORD REFLEXES

Barry D. Goldstein

TABLE OF CONTENTS

I.   Introduction 36

II.   Background 36
         A.   Ventral Root Responses 36
               1.   Monosynaptic Reflex 36
               2.   Polysynaptic Reflex (PSR) 36
         B.   Dorsal Root Responses 36
               1.   Dorsal Root Potential 38
               2.   Dorsal Root Reflex 38

III.   Toxicology of Spinal Cord Reflexes 38
         A.   Chemical Agents 38
         B.   Drugs 41

IV.   Methodology 41
         A.   General Procedures 41
               1.   In Vivo 41
               2.   In Vitro 42
         B.   Stimulating and Recording Techniques 42
               1.   In Vivo 42
               2.   In Vitro 43
         C.   Measurement of Potentials 44
         D.   Monosynaptic Reflex Testing Protocols 44
               1.   Excitation 44
               2.   Inhibition 46
         E.   Dorsal Root Responses 47

V.   Summary 48

Acknowledgment 48

References 48

I. INTRODUCTION

The spinal cord is the gateway to and from the central nervous system (CNS). The spinal cord is the first place that sensory input is processed and in most cases the last place motor output is processed. The motor output is through the alpha-motoneuron and therefore as quoted by Sherington; "is the final common pathway within the CNS". Thus, the study of spinal cord function following toxic insult is very important.

This chapter deals with spinal cord reflexes. In particular, the methods used to study both excitatory and inhibitory pathways and how these methods can and are used in toxicological research.

II. BACKGROUND

Studies on spinal cord reflexes can tell us about the condition of the motoneuron, the central terminal of the primary afferent neuron, and interneurons. However, all of these neuronal substrates cannot be studied using only one method. Some of the methods entail variations of monosynaptic reflex (MSR) testing, some entail the study of polysynaptic reflexes (PSR), and other methods entail the study of primary afferent depolarization (PAD).

A. Ventral Root Responses
1. Monosynaptic Reflex (MSR)

The MSR is a two-neuron arc (Figure 1) arising from group Ia afferents (muscle spindle primary endings) and terminating on homonymous alpha-motoneurons. It is a compound action potential recorded in the ventral roots following activation by either stretch or direct stimulation of a muscle nerve or stimulation of the dorsal root and is directly proportional to the size of the motoneuron pool.[42] The actual potential recorded reflects what is known as the discharge zone.[42] Figure 2 shows the unconditioned MSR, which represents the discharge zone of the motoneuronal pool. This particular MSR is activated by stimulation of the dorsal roots and recorded from the ventral roots. This same afferent volley will also excite but not cause the firing of other motoneuron pools. That pool of motoneurons is known as the subliminal fringe.[18] Tetanic stimulation of the afferent nerve recruits the subliminal fringe such that a potentiation of the MSR occurs (Figure 2). This is known as post-tetanic potentiation (PTP).[43] The percent increase in the PTP is a measure of the viability of the discharge zone and its subliminal fringes.[20,21] Therefore, any change in the amplitude or area of the unconditioned MSR or PTP may be indicative of depression or facilitation in the spinal cord.

MSR testing can be used to study excitatory as well as inhibitory activity in the spinal cord. The inhibitory responses include postsynaptic, presynaptic, and recurrent inhibition.[21] Figure 1 is a schematic diagram of the different types of responses obtainable from the ventral root recording.

2. Polysynaptic Reflex (PSR)

The PSR is an asynchronous discharge which immediately follows the MSR in time course (Figure 2). It is evoked by proprioceptive as well as cutaneous primary afferents and has been attributed to the afferent fibers conducting in the 35 to 72 m/sec range.[41] Changes in the PSR can be an indication of changes in interneuronal activity and/or smaller-diameter sensory fiber input.

B. Dorsal Root Responses

The dorsal root responses discussed in this chapter have been shown to be reflections of primary afferent depolarization and presynaptic inhibition.[40,48]

Monosynaptic Reflex

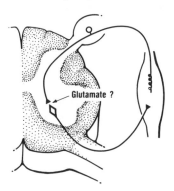

Postsynaptic Inhibition

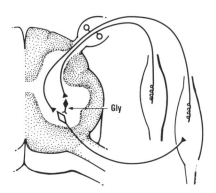

Presynaptic Inhibition

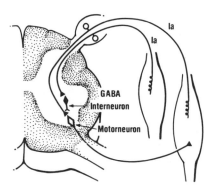

Recurrent Inhibition

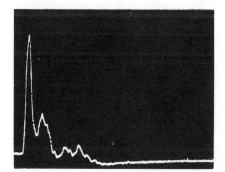

FIGURE 1.   Schematic diagram of four different reflex pathways in the spinal cord.

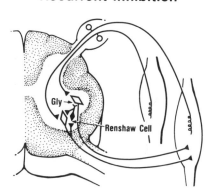

0.5mv
2.0ms

FIGURE 2.   Oscilloscope tracing of the monosynaptic (MSR) and polysynaptic (PSR) reflex discharge (left) and the post-tetanic potentiation (PTP) of that response (right). The MSR is the synchronous volley on the left which is followed by the PSR. The PTP was elicited by stimulating the L_7 dorsal root at 500 Hz for 10 sec.

These responses (infra vide) were first described by Barron and Matthews.[1,2] However, it was not until Frank and Fourtes[27] showed that test stimuli to the hamstring muscle-nerve reduced the excitatory postsynaptic potential (EPSP) in medial gastrocnemious motoneurons by 50% that it became clear that presynaptic inhibition occurred.[23,24] This was followed by a series of experiments which showed that primary afferent terminals could be depolarized and was, in fact, responsible for presynaptic inhibition.[26] Following these classical studies it was further recognized that the antidromic potentials first recorded by Baron and Matthews[1] were actually reflections of primary afferent terminal depolarization (PAD) and presynaptic inhibition. The pharmacology of PAD has been thoroughly investigated and reviewed.[39] It is now clear that PAD is mediated in part by a GABA in interneuron.

1. Dorsal Root Potential (DRP)

The DRP is an antidromic, nonpropagating, electrotonic potential. It was first recorded by Barron and Matthews[1] and later labeled DRP_I-DRP_v by Lloyd and McIntyre.[44] Lloyd's DRP_v corresponds to the DRP recorded by Barron and Matthews[1] and seen in Figure 5. The DRP is a population potential and is made up of hundreds of smaller depolarizations in single afferent terminals. It must be understood that changes in the area of the DRP reflect changes in the depolarization of hundreds of primary afferent terminals.

2. Dorsal Root Reflex (DRR)

The DRR is an antidromic, propagating compound action potential which can be recorded in dorsal roots (see Figure 5)[1,5,25] and/or peripheral nerves.[51,52] Some investigators believe that the DRR is the result of the rising phase of the DRP.[22] However, there is no DRR generated from brainstem-evoked DRPs.[7,56] Thus, it is unclear as to where the DRR is initiated. It does seem to be a good indication of phasic PAD and is very sensitive to drugs affecting GABA transmission.[39]

III. TOXICOLOGY OF SPINAL CORD REFLEXES

There are two major types of studies of the effects of toxins on spinal cord reflex function. The first involves the use of toxins as tools to delineate out the physiology and pharmacology of the reflex pathways.[13,14] For instance, picrotoxin, bicuculline, and stychnine are toxins which specifically affect GABA and glycine neurotransmission.[13-15,17,39] These toxins are all known convulsants or CNS stimulants. They are used routinely in the study of these type of synapses. The second involves the use of toxins which have no specific action as do the above agents, i.e., they produce a dysfunction as a result of axonal damage, membrane damage, or any kind of nonspecific effect. Due to the many reviews of the spinal cord action of the toxins in the first category,[13,14,17,39] this chapter will only review the effects of the toxins in the second category.

There have only been a few studies on spinal cord function following toxic insult. Most of these involve agents which produce neuropathies of one kind or another.[10-12,34,36,46,49] These chemicals and drugs usually produce neurological sequalae which include ataxia and loss of tendon reflexes. Most of the studies have been performed on ventral root responses, in particular, the monosynaptic reflex (MSR) since this spinal cord reflex is involved in proprioceptive function. There are only two studies which have examined effects on dorsal root responses.

The toxicological studies on spinal cord reflexes can be divided into two major categories: chemical agents and drugs.

A. Chemical Agents

There are several agents which have been studied which have in common the production of giant axonal swellings. These include acrylamide,[46] the hexacarbons,[45,49] and IDPN.[10-12,34,36]

Acrylamide is a vinyl monomer which has been shown to produce distal giant axonal swellings.[46] The effects of acrylamide on spinal cord reflexes have been extensively investigated.[19,29-32] These studies have shown several things: (1) the MSR is depressed following chronic administration of ACR, (2) the DRP and DRR are depressed following chronic administration, and (3) the MSR and DRR are facilitated following acute administration of ACR.

The depressed MSR appears to be the result of damage to the primary afferent terminal as shown by studying (1) changes in electrical excitability (PTP),[29] (2) changes in input-output,[30] (3) changes in repetitive stimulation (apparent transmitter turnover parameters),[30] and (4) changes in drug-induced excitability.[32]

Goldstein and Lowndes[29] found that while the unconditioned MSR was depressed, the maximally potentiated MSR (PTP) was normal, suggesting that the motoneurons were responding normally but that the primary afferent terminals (PAT) were not. This was strengthened by showing that the critical input necessary to produce a threshold MSR was increased, i.e., more PAT were necessary to activate the MSR, and that replenishment of the transmitter in the PAT was depressed.[30] There was one problem with the explanation of these data. It was all based on indirect data suggesting the motoneuron was normal at the time of the experiment since the changes in the PAT were studied through ventral root responses. Therefore, another study was performed to determine whether the excitability of the motoneuron to quipazine, a serotonin agonist, was altered following chronic ACR administration.[32] It was found that the spontaneous discharge of the motoneuron responded in a dose-dependent manner to quipazine and that there was no change in this dose-response in the ACR-treated groups (Figure 3). However, the dose-response relationship of the MSR to quipazine was significantly depressed following ACR administration (Figure 4). These data suggest that the PAT are the site of dysfunction early in the time course of the neuropathy.

In a recent preliminary study an attempt was made to further characterize the effects of ACR on the PAT.[19] It was found that following chronic administration of ACR the DRP could not be evoked even at stimulation intensities as great as 90 V. These data further support the studies on the MSR following chronic administration of ACR.

A paradoxical effect is observed when ACR is administered acutely.[31] Goldstein and Fincher have shown that as early as 30 min following a single injection of 50 mg/kg ACR, the MSR and DRR are significantly increased in area and amplitude.[31] This action on the spinal reflexes is as yet unexplained.

There have been no experimental studies of spinal cord reflexes in hexacarbon neuropathy. However, there has been a clinical study of the H-reflex.[4] In that study, they found the humans exposed to *n*-hexane had facilitated H-reflexes suggesting increased excitability of the motoneuron. This effect does not correspond with the changes observed with ACR and therefore need to be studied more carefully in an experimental model.

IDPN, unlike acrylamide and the hexacarbons, produces axonal swellings proximal to the soma of the motoneuron.[10-12,34,36] Gold and Lowndes[28] have found that the MSR in animals treated with IDPN is significantly reduced. Furthermore, MSR testing of recurrent inhibition in IDPN-treated animals shows a significant reduction to about 50% of control. This suggests that the proximal swellings adversely affect not only normal excitability but also inhibition.

Organophosphorous (OP) agents also affect spinal cord reflexes[33,37,50,54,55] Several studies have been performed with different OP agents administered over different time periods. They have all found that the MSR and DRR are depressed following OP administration. This includes studies on delayed neurotoxicity resulting from TOCP administration,[37] acute administration of soman, sarin, and tabun[50,54,55] and subacute administration of soman and sarin.[33] It should be noted that the mechanism of the effects of these agents on the spinal

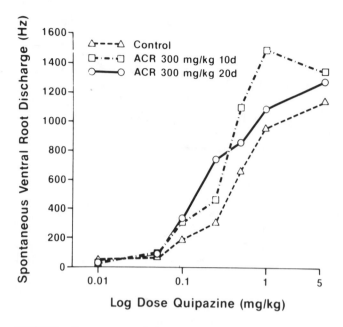

FIGURE 3.   Dose-response relationships between quipazine and the spontaneous ventral root discharge in control, ACR 10, and ACR 20 cats. The pre-quipazine frequency was substracted from each point.

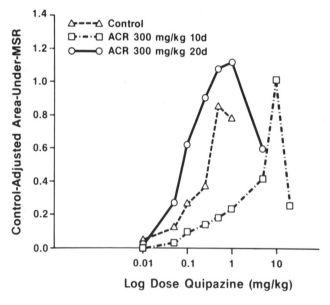

FIGURE 4.   Dose-response relationships between quipazine and the area-under-the-monosynaptic reflex in control, ACR 10, and ACR 20 cats. The pre-quipazine area was subtracted from each point.

reflexes are probably entirely different. The delayed neurotoxicity is probably a nonspecific effect due to nerve degeneration. The acute and subacute effects of the OP agents on spinal reflexes is probably the result of enzyme inhibition or even some direct effect of the agent. There is no evidence which suggests that the doses used in the soman and sarin studies cause a delayed neurotoxicity.

The herbicide 2-ethyl-4-ethylamino-6-methoxy-S-triazine (EEM) has been shown to facilitate the MSR, the PSR, and the DRR in spinal cord transected animals. However, in intact animals anesthetized with chloralose, the PSR and DRR were depressed.[9] It thus appears that EEM acts at both segmental as well as suprasegmental sites to cause its effects. The actions at suprasegmental sites probably overide any action at the spinal cord level.

B. Drugs

Spinal cord reflexes have been studied following administration of several different drugs. The most studied of these drugs is ethanol. Ethanol depresses the MSR[38] and augments the DRP.[15] The MSR in spinal cord transected animals has been shown to decrease in a dose-dependent manner following ethanol administration.[47] This has also been shown to occur in unanesthetized rabbits when studying the H-reflex.[8] The decrease in the MSR is accompanied by an increase in the DRP and primary afferent depolarization (PAD).[47] These changes correspond to each other and can partially explain why ethanol causes ataxia and loss of reflexes. The increase in PAD will cause a decrease in the MSR through presynaptic inhibition.

IV. METHODOLOGY

This section will describe in detail both in vivo and in vitro techniques used to determine spinal cord reflex activity following toxic insult.

The animal models used to study reflex actions in the spinal cord include cat, rat, and frog. The most extensive work in vivo has been performed in the cat. Therefore, the in vivo methods described below only mention the cat as the animal model. The rat is a good model for short term studies but usually cannot be maintained very long during the experimental procedure due to the combination of toxic insult, spinal shock, and extensive surgery.

The in vitro model is the isolated, hemisected frog spinal cord. In vitro techniques afford the ability to alter the ionic makeup of the extracellular environment and the ability to perform DC recordings of the spinal reflexes, which becomes important when studying baseline changes in polarization.

A. General Procedures
1. In Vivo

Spinal cord reflex studies have been performed on both anesthetized and unanesthetized, spinal cord-transected cats. It is recommended that unanesthetized spinal cord-transected cats be used since general anesthetics are synaptic depressants and could affect the system being studied.

Adult cats weighing 2 to 4 kg are pretreated with atropine methylnitrate (1.0 mg/kg i.p.) and initially anesthetized with diethyl ether. The methylatropine inhibits bronchiole secretions which occur as a result of the ether. A tracheal cannula is inserted and the animal is mechanically respired with a mixture of room air and ether. The mixture is adjusted for the proper depth of anesthesia. The carotid arteries are ligated and a bilateral vagotomy is performed. A cannula is inserted into one of the carotids to monitor blood pressure. This is used to determine the physiological state of the animal. If the mean blood pressure falls below 60 mmHg, the experiment is terminated and the data discarded. The spinal cord is transected at the atlanto-occipital junction (C_1). A midline incision is made along the dorsal aspect of the neck. The muscles are separated along their fascial planes and the cisterna magna isolated. The dura is opened and the spinal cord transected. The wound is packed with saline-soaked gauze and closed. The ether is removed and the animal is mechanically respired throughout the experiment. A vertebral artery clamp is placed over the dorsal aspect of the neck for about 15 min. Clamping of the vertebral arteries along with the ligation of the carotid arteries causes brain ischemia. Therefore, the only viable portion of the CNS is the spinal cord (as long as the animal is respired). A venous cannula is then placed in the antecubetal vein for injection of drugs. Gallamine triethiodide (2 mg/kg) is administered intravenously as needed to prevent abnormal muscular movements resulting from the spinal cord transection.

A dorsal laminectomy is performed from vertebral segments L_3 to S_2. The dura mater is incised longitudinally and the spinal cord exposed. The spinal roots L_6 to S_1 are bilaterally isolated and the ventral roots cut proximal to where they enter the dura mater. The dorsal roots can be left intact for peripheral nerve stimulation or they can be cut proximal to where they enter the dura mater for spinal nerve stimulation. The nerves on the contralateral side are cut to assure that no peripheral sensory input affects the reflexes studied.

The peripheral nerves used most often in these studies are the quadriceps, biceps-semi-tendinosus, posterior biceps semitendinosus, medial and lateral gastrocnemious, soleus, and the sural. They can all be isolated in the hindlimb through the popliteal fossa.

If peripheral nerves are isolated, surgical pins are inserted at the knee and ankle so that the leg can be kept rigid. The animal is placed in a spinal unit and the skin flaps from both surgical cavities are tied back to make oil pools. The cavities are filled with mineral oil and maintained at 37°C. The temperature of the cord should be carefully monitored since changes in temperature can significantly alter the excitability of the recorded potentials.[21]

2. In Vitro

In vitro techniques include the study of spinal reflex activity in isolated, hemisected frog spinal cord. *Rana pipiens* or *Rana catesbiana* are used in these experiments.

The animal is cooled on ice for at least 1 hr to assure anesthesia and is kept on ice during the surgery. The spinal cord is isolated by dorsal laminectomy and the lumbar cord removed with the spinal roots intact. The cord is placed in a cooled dish with circulating Ringer solution. The cord is hemisected sagittally and half of the cord with dorsal and ventral roots isolated is placed in a recording chamber. The temperature of the bath is maintained at about 22°C.

The amphibian Ringer solution should have the following composition: NaCl, 100 mM, KCl, 2.5 mM; Na_2HPO_4, 2.5 mM; NaH_2PO_4, 0.45 mM, $CaCl_2$, 1.9 mM, $NaHCO_3$, 12 mM, glucose, 2.8 mM. It is equilibrated with 95% O_2/5% CO_2 and the pH maintained at 7.4.[15]

B. Stimulating and Recording Techniques

1. In Vivo

The ventral root (L_7 or S_1) is placed on a bipolar platinum wire recording electrode (shielded, 26 to 28 gauge wire) for recording the MSR. If the DRP and DRR are to be recorded simultaneously, then the adjacent dorsal root or a piece of the adjacent dorsal root is placed on another recording electrode. The electrode recording the DRP should be very close to the dorsal root entry zone since it is an electronic potential. Figure 5 shows the electrode placement for recording the MSR, DRP, and DRR. In Figure 5, the L_7 dorsal root is placed on a stimulating electrode for the recording of the above potentials. However, these potentials can also be elicited by stimulating any of the perpheral nerves mentioned above. The potentials are elicited by stimulating the appropriate nerve with square wave pulses of 0.05 to 0.2 msec duration at the required intensity at a rate no faster than every 5 sec (0.2 Hz). Any faster rate will cause the potentials to be variable in size due to insufficient replenishment of transmitter at the ready-releasable site. The required intensity depends upon what fiber types you want contributing to the recorded potentials. For example, if you only want group Ia input, which will elicit the MSR, DRP, and DRR (not PSR) then the stimulus intensity should be 1.4× threshold. If you want to add the PSR, then the stimulus intensity would have to be great enough to include group II and smaller fibers. Therefore, at least 4 to 6× threshold for group II and greater for group III and IV (equivalent to C-fiber intensity

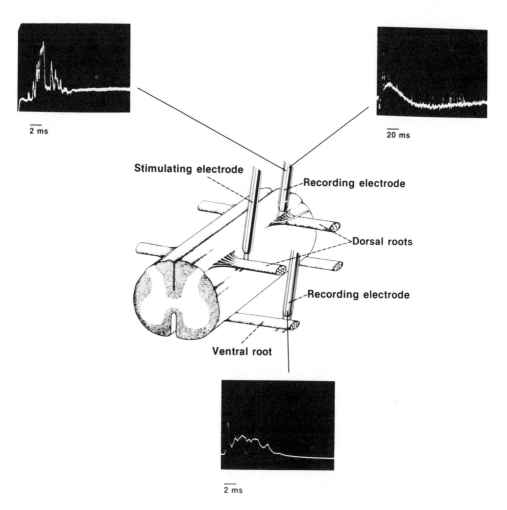

FIGURE 5. Electrode placement for recording of MSR, DRR, and DRP. Top trace on left is the DRR. Top trace of right is the DRP and the bottom trace is the MSR.

should be used). If all that is needed is a maximal response, then ten times the threshold (or supramaximal) intensity should be used.

The recording electrode is coupled to a preamplifier (AC, bandpass 0.3 Hz to 30 kHz). The amplified signals are shunted to an oscilloscope for display. For measurement purposes, the recorded potentials can either be photographed off the oscilloscope with a Polaroid camera or a kymograph camera or if a computer or signal averager is available (this is preferred) the potentials can be acquired and averaged.

2. In Vitro

There are several ways to stimulate and record DC potentials in vitro. One of the best ways is with suction electrodes. The dorsal and ventral roots are drawn up into fluid filled suction electrodes. The electrode on one dorsal root is connected to a stimulator and the other two electrodes, one on the ventral root and one on an adjacent dorsal root, are connected to DC amplifiers. The DC potentials are displayed on an oscilloscope and the baseline activity (DC level) can be continuously recorded with a linear recorder. The evoked potentials (MSR and DRP) can be photographed or acquired and averaged as described above.

C. Measurement of Potentials

Once the MSR, PSR, DRP, and/or DRR are acquired, as mentioned above, there are several different ways to measure them. These include measurement of amplitude, area, and/or both.

Amplitude measurement can only be performed with MSR potentials. The reason is that it is the only synchronous response in the spinal cord. The other responses are either asynchronous (PSR and DRR) or slow and broad (DRP). The amplitude measurement is simply performed by measuring the peak height of the MSR and adjusting it for the amplification factor used when it was recorded. If it is not adjusted, then the measurement is meaningless.

Area measurement can be used to analyze all of the potentials mentioned above. Since these potentials are population potentials the area under the curve would be a better indicator of what is happening to the entire population and thus a better way of analyzing these potentials. There are several ways in which area can be measured. This is dependent upon how the potentials were acquired. If the potentials were photographed, then the waveforms can be cut out of the paper and weighed on a balance or a planimeter can be used. If a computer or signal averager is available then the potentials can be integrated. Again, the areas determined must be adjusted for the amplification so that all the potentials are normalized.

The best way to analyze some of these potentials is to measure both amplitude and area since it is possible that the area under the curve will change but the amplitude will not and vice versa. A way to combine area with amplitude is to determine the ratio of the change in amplitude over the area.

D. Monosynaptic Reflex Testing Protocols

All of the spinal cord potentials described above can be used to study neurotoxic insult to the spinal cord. The one problem with using these particular techniques is that the interpretation as to the site of action of the toxin can be misleading. Changes in these potentials can be indicative of alterations in the primary afferent terminal, an interneuron, the motoneuron, or any combination of these neuronal substrates. It is, therefore, important to understand the limitations of the techniques used in studying spinal cord function.

There are many different protocols using the MSR as a tool for the study of spinal cord function. These protocols have been reviewed elsewhere.[21] However, for the sake of clarity, they will be reviewed again in this chapter.

1. Excitation

The first thing to study in MSR testing is the unconditioned response. It is important to know whether a toxin affects the normal response of the MSR following dorsal root or peripheral nerve stimulation. This is performed by simply comparing the unconditioned MSR in control and treated animals.

Following this procedure several tests of excitability can be performed. These include post-tetanic potentiation (PTP), repetitive synaptic activation, input-output relationships, and alterations in dose-response curves to known drugs which increase motoneuron excitability.

PTP, as mentioned in the background, is an enhancement of neurotransmission following tetanic stimulation. It can be used as an indicator of MSR excitability. Stimulation of a peripheral nerve or the dorsal roots at anywhere from 50 to 500 Hz for 10 to 15 sec causes a considerable increase in the MSR. This conditioned response is one way in which a determination of site of action can be made. For example, Goldstein and Lowndes[29] have shown that the unconditioned MSR is depressed following acrylamide administration but the PTP of the MSR appears normal. This suggests that all the motoneurons present can respond to neurotransmitter activation but the primary afferent terminal in the resting state does not activate the appropriate number of motoneurons. Conversely, it is possible that the

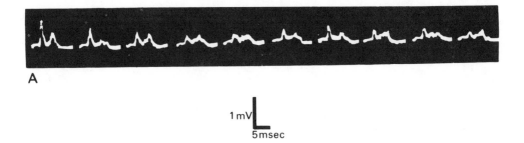

A

1 mV

5 msec

FIGURE 6.   Homosynaptic depression observed in a normal cat. Stimulus frequency was 2 Hz.

resting MSR and the conditioned MSR (via PTP) are depressed. This would suggest that the motoneuron is not responding properly to an input volley. The time course of the return to resting state would be another important piece of information. It would tell how long this excitability lasted.

Repetitive synaptic activation can be used as an indicator of release, mobilization, and replenishment of neurotransmitter at the group Ia — motoneuronal synapse.[6] Activating the MSR with a train of ten stimuli at 2, 5, and 10 Hz causes a progressive decline in its amplitude. This decline has been defined as homosynaptic depression (Figure 6).[3] From this decline, apparent transmitter turnover parameters of release and replenishment can be estimated.[6,30] To carry out this procedure, the MSR has to be recorded during a train of ten stimuli at 2, 5, and 10 Hz. The amplitudes of the MSR are determined and expressed as a fraction of the first response in the train (Figure 7). The constant fraction of transmitter released and replenished is determined using the following formulae:

$$p = \frac{(1 - Q_t)(1 - Qss)}{(1 - Qss) - (Qss(1 - Q_t))}$$

and,

$$r = \frac{1}{t} - \ln \frac{1 - Qss}{1 - Qss(1 - p)}$$

where p = constant fraction of transmitter released, Q_t = the amplitude of the second pulse in the train, Qss = the average amplitude of the plateau, r = the constant rate of replenishment of transmitter, and t = the frequency of stimulation.

Input-output relationships give an indication of the amount of presynaptic volley (number of afferent fibers) necessary to produce a liminal motoneuronal response.[6,21,30] This can be used as an indicator of whether there is the appropriate amount of presynaptic volley to produce a threshold response. This is performed by recording the incoming volley from the appropriate dorsal root and recording the corresponding ventral root response. First, the maximal ventral root response is recorded along with the corresponding dorsal root response. These responses are defined as unity. Next, the stimulus intensity is reduced in a sequential manner and both the dorsal root and ventral root responses are recorded. This is done until the ventral root response disappears. The amplitude of the dorsal and ventral root responses are then expressed as a fraction of the corresponding unity response and the input (dorsal root responses) is plotted against the output (ventral root responses). Figure 8 shows the relationship of the input to the output of the MSR evoked from the soleus nerve in normal and acrylamide-treated cats. As seen, there is a linear relationship between input and output. Extrapolation to the zero output gives you the critical input (Qc). The critical input is the amount of afferent input necessary to produce a threshold output (supra vide).

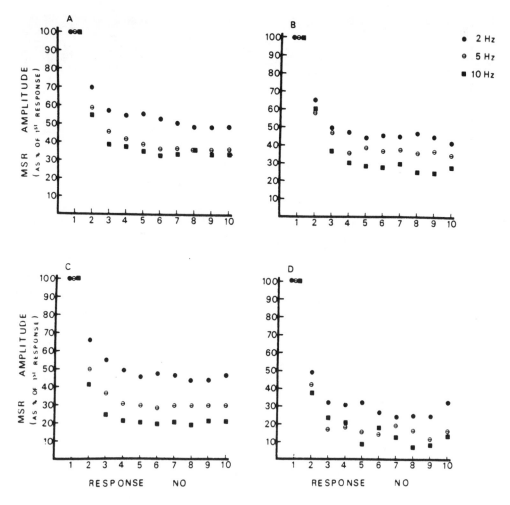

FIGURE 7. Homosynaptic depression of amplitude of the monosynaptic response in normal cats and cats with acrylamide neuropathy. A train of 10 pulses was applied to the soleus nerve and recorded in the ventral root at 2, 5, or 10 Hz. Ordinate is amplitude of MSR relative to the first response in train. Abscissa is response number. (A) Normal cats; (B) 75 mg/kg acrylamide; (C) 150 mg/kg acrylamide; (D) 300 mg/kg acrylamide. Values are means without SEM.

Drugs can be used to alter the excitability of the MSR so that changes in the evoked responses can be compared in normal and neurotoxin-impaired animals. The alpha-moto-neuron responds to many neurotransmitters due to descending control of the spinal cord.[17] One of these is serotonin. Generation of dose-response curves to a serotonin agonist will show progressive increases in the MSR area and amplitude.[32] Comparisons can then be made of the excitability changes of the motoneuron.[32] Figures 3 and 4 show the dose-response curves generated by increasing doses of quipazine, a serotonin agonist.

2. Inhibition

Inhibition can also be determined using MSR testing.[21] As mentioned briefly above, test stimuli to appropriate muscle nerves, will set up inhibitory responses at the motoneuron. These inhibitory responses are measured as a decrease area or amplitude of the MSR. The inhibitory responses which can be measured are recurrent, postsynaptic, and presynaptic inhibition. (See Figure 1 for schematic representation.)

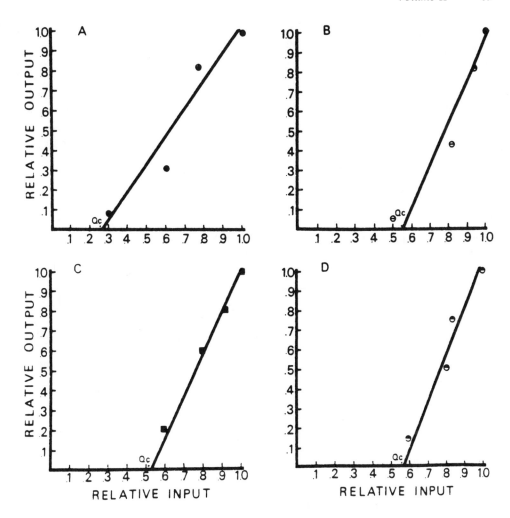

FIGURE 8. Input-output relationship of the soleus-ventral root MSR pathway in normal and acrylamide-treated cats. Ordinate is the amplitude of the ventral root compound action potential (CAP) response relative to the supramaximal ventral root CAP. Abscissa is amplitude of dorsal root CAP response relative to supramaximal dorsal root CAP. Qc is the critical input. (A) Normal cat; (B) cat given 75 mg/kg acrylamide; (C) cat given 150 mg/kg acrylamide; (D) cat given 300 mg/kg acrylamide. See text for further explanation of methods. Qc was significantly elevated in cats administered 75 and 300, but not 150 mg/kg acrylamide.

The techniques for the measurement of these three types of inhibition are basically the same. The only difference is the nerve which is used as the conditioning stimulus. Once the MSR is recorded, conditioning stimuli are presented to the appropriate nerve at fixed intervals of 5 to 1000 msec prior to the test stimuli to the dorsal root or another muscle nerve. The decrease in the MSR spike as a result of the conditioning stimulus is plotted against the interval between the conditioning and test stimuli. These curves can then be used to ascertain any differences in neurotoxin-treated animals.

E. Dorsal Root Responses

Studies on doral root responses, i.e., the DRP and DRR can be carried out simultaneously with the studies of the MSR and PSR. The protocols for the study of dorsal root responses include the determination of area under the curve, input-output relationships, and excitability changes.

The protocols described above are basically similar to those described for MSR testing.

The differences are that changes in the area under a DRP may be indicative of several phenomena. For example, a depressed DRP may actually be a depolarized primary afferent terminal, an inhibited release of transmitter from the interneuron or the stimulated primary afferent, or it could be a decreased responsiveness of the postsynaptic primary afferent terminal. These changes have to be studied in relation to the effects on the DRR or in vitro where DC recordings can show changes in terminal polarization. If the DRP decreases and the DRR increases, this suggests a depolarization. If they are both depressed, it suggests that there is a dysfunction either pre- or postsynaptically. In vitro studies utilizing isolated frog spinal cord with DC recordings[15] can best determine the exact nature of the effects of the toxin on this system.

V. SUMMARY

In summary, this chapter has described some of the electrophysiological techniques used to study functional changes in spinal cord reflexes. There are many other techniques which can be used to study spinal cord reflex activity[24-26] and as the field expands I am sure more and more of these techniques will be employed.

ACKNOWLEDGMENTS

The author wishes to thank Ms. Sandra Usry for her typing of this manuscript. This review, as well as, some of the cited research was supported by the U.S. Army Medical Research and Development Command DAMD17-82-C-2217 and NIH grant NS-18664 from NINCDS.

REFERENCES

1. **Barron, D. H. and Matthews, B. H. C.,** Intermittent conduction in the spinal cord, *J. Physiol.,* 85, 73, 1935.
2. **Barron, D. H. and Matthews, B. H. C.,** The interpretation of potential changes in the spinal cord, *J. Physiol.,* 92, 276, 1938.
3. **Beswick, F. B. and Evanson, J. M.,** Homosynaptic depression of the monosynaptic reflex following its activation, *J. Physiol.,* 135, 400, 1957.
4. **Barvaccio, F., Ammendola, A., Barruffo, L., and Carlomagno, S.,** H-reflex behavior in glue (N-hexane) neuropathy, *Clin. Toxicol.,* 18(12), 1369, 1981.
5. **Brooks, C. M. and Koizumi, K.,** Origin of the dorsal root reflex, *J. Neurophysiol.,* 19, 61, 1956.
6. **Capek, R. and Esplin, B.,** Homosynaptic depression and transmitter turnover in spinal monosynaptic pathway, *J. Neurophysiol.,* 40, 95, 1977.
7. **Carpenter, D., Engberg, I., and Lundberg, A.,** Primary afferent depolarization evoked from brainstem and cerebellum, *Arch. Ital. Biol.,* 104, 73, 1966.
8. **Chandran, A. P., Marya, R. K., and Maini, B. K.,** Effect of ethanol on H-reflex in unanesthetized rabbits, *Physiol. Behav.,* 26, 967, 1981.
9. **Chiba, S.,** Inhibition of spinal polysynaptic reflex and augmentation of muscle contraction by 2-ethyl-4-ethylamino-6-methoxy-S-triazine, *Jpn. J. Pharmac.,* 19, 451, 1969.
10. **Chou, S. M. and Hartmann, H. A.,** Axonal lesions and waltzing syndrome after IDPN administration in rats. With a concept — ''Axostasis'', *Acta Neuropathol.,* 3, 428, 1964.
11. **Chou, S. M. and Hartmann, H. A.,** Electronmicroscopy of focal neuroaxonal lesions produced by β,β'-iminodipropionitrile (IDPN) in rats, *Acta Neuropathol.,* 4, 590, 1965.
12. **Clark, A. W., Griffin, J. W., and Price, D. L.,** The axonal pathology in chronic IDPN intoxication, *J. Neuropathol. Exp. Neurol.,* 39, 42, 1980.
13. **Curtis, D. R.,** The pharmacology of central and peripheral inhibition, *Pharmacol. Rev.,* 15, 333, 1963.
14. **Curtis, D. R.,** The pharmacology of spinal postsynaptic inhibition, *Prog. Brain Res.,* 31, 171, 1969.

15. **Davidoff, R. A.,** The effects of bicuculline on the isolated spinal cord of the frog, *Exp. Neurol.,* 35, 179, 1972.
16. **Davidoff, R. A.,** Alcohol and presynaptic inhibition in an isolated spinal cord preparation, *Arch. Neurol.,* 28, 60, 1973.
17. **Davidoff, R. A.,** *Handbook of the Spinal Cord,* Vol. 1, Marcel Dekker, New York, 1983.
18. **Denny-Brown, D. E. and Sherrington, E. S.,** Subliminal fringe in spinal flexion, *J. Physiol.,* 66, 175, 1928.
19. **DeRojas, T. and Goldstein, B. D.,** Acrylamide alters the function of the primary afferent terminal, *Soc. Neuroscience Abstr.,* 12, 995, 1985.
20. **Esplin, D. W.,** Criteria for assessing effects of depressant drugs on spinal cord synaptic transmission, with examples of drug selectivity (1), (2), *Arch. Int. Pharmacodynam.,* 143, 479, 1963.
21. **Esplin, D. W.,** *Synaptic System Models in Experimental Models of Epilepsy,* Purpura, D. P., Penry, J. K., Tower, D. B., Woodbury, D. M., and Walter, R. D., Eds., Raven Press, New York, 1972, 223.
22. **Eccles, J. C. and Malcolm, J. L.,** Dorsal root potentials of the spinal cord, *J. Neurophysiol.,* 9, 139, 1946.
23. **Eccles, J. C., Eccles, R. M., and Magni, F.,** Presynaptic inhibition in the spinal cord, *J. Physiol.,* 154, 28P, 1960.
24. **Eccles, J. C., Eccles, R. M., and Magni, F.,** Central inhibitory action attributable to presynaptic depolarization produced by muscle afferent volleys, *J. Physiol.,* 159, 147, 1961.
25. **Eccles, J. C., Kozak, W., and Magni, F.,** Dorsal root reflexes of muscle group 1 afferent fibres, *J. Physiol.,* 159, 128, 1961.
26. **Eccles, J. C., Magni, F., and Willis, W. D.,** Depolarization of central terminals of group I afferent fibers from muscle, *J. Physiol.,* 160, 62, 1962.
27. **Frank, K. and Fourtes, M. G. F.,** Presynaptic and postsynaptic inhibition of monosynaptic reflexes, *Fed. Proc.,* 16, 39, 1957.
28. **Gold, B. G. and Lowndes, H. E.,** Electrophysiological investigation of β,β′-imminodiproprionitrile neurotoxicity: monosynaptic reflexes and recurrent inhibition, *Neurotoxicology,* 5, 1, 1984.
29. **Goldstein, B. D. and Lowndes, H. E.,** Spinal cord defect in the peripheral neuropathy resulting from acrylamide, *Neurotoxicology,* 1, 75, 1979.
30. **Goldstein, B. D. and Lowndes, H. E.,** Group Ia primary afferent terminal defect in cats with acrylamide neuropathy, *Neurotoxicology,* 2, 297, 1981.
31. **Goldstein, B. D. and Fincher, D. R.,** Paradoxical changes in spinal cord reflexes following the acute administration of acrylamide, *Toxicol. Lett.,* 31, 93, 1986.
32. **Goldstein, B. D.,** Paradoxical changes in Spinal cord reflexes following the acute administration of acrylamide, *Toxicol. Lett.,* 31, 93, 1986.
33. **Goldstein, B. D. and Fincher, D. R.,** Soman depresses the spinal monosynaptic reflex without producing a delayed neurotoxicity, *Toxicologist,* 5, 86, 1985.
34. **Griffin, J. W. and Price, D. L.,** Proximal axonopathies induced by toxic chemicals, in *Experimental and Clinical Neurotoxicology,* Spencer, P. S. and Schaumburg, H. H., Eds., Baltimore, Williams & Wilkins, Baltimore, 1980, 161.
35. **Griffin, J. W., Price, D. L., and Drachman, D. B.,** Impaired axonal regeneration in acrylamide intoxication, *J. Neurobiol.,* 8, 355, 1977.
36. **Griffin, J. W., Gold, B. G., Cork, L. C., Price, D. L., and Lowndes, H. E.,** IDPN neuropathy in the cat: coexistence of proximal and distal axonal swellings, *Neuropathol. Appl. Neurobiol.,* 8, 351, 1982.
37. **Lapadula, D. M., Kinnes, C. G., Somjen, G. G., and Abou-donia, M. B.,** Monosynaptic reflex depression in cats with organophosphorous neuropathy; effects of tri-o-cresyl phosphate, *Neurotoxicology,* 3, 51, 1982.
38. **Lathers, C. M. and Smith, C. M.,** Ethanol effects on muscle spindle afferent activity and spinal reflexes, *J. Pharmacol. Exp. Ther.,* 197, 126, 1976.
39. **Levy, R. A.,** The role of GABA in primary afferent depolarization, *Prog. Neurobiol.,* 9, 211, 1977.
40. **Levy, R. A.,** Presynaptic control of input to the central nervous system, *Can. J. Physiol. Pharmacol.,* 58, 751, 1980.
41. **Lloyd, D. P. C.,** Neuron patterns controlling transmission of ipsilateral hindlimb reflexes in the cat, *J. Neurophysiol.,* 6, 293, 1943.
42. **Lloyd, D. P. C.,** On the relationship between discharge zone and subliminal fringe in a motoneuron pool supplied by a homogenous presynaptic pathway, *Yale J. Biol. Med.,* 18, 117, 1945.
43. **Lloyd, D. P. C.,** Post-tetanic potentiation of response in monosynaptic reflex pathways of the spinal cord, *J. Gen. Physiol.,* 33, 147, 1949.
44. **Lloyd, D. P. C. and McIntyre, A. K.,** On the origin of dorsal root potentials, *J. Gen. Physiol.,* 32, 409, 1949.
45. **Mendell, J. R., Saida, K., Ganansia, M. F., Jackson, D. B., Weiss, H., Gardinier, R. W., Christman, C., Allen, N., Couri, D., O'Neill, J., Marks, B., and Hetland, L.,** Toxic polyneuropathy produced by methyl-*n*-butyl ketone, *Science,* 185, 787, 1974.

46. **Prineas, J.,** The pathogenesis of dying-back polyneuropathies. II. An ultrastructural study of experimental acrylamide intoxication in the cat, *Neurobiology,* 28, 598, 1969.
47. **Rinaldi, P. C., Nishurma, L. Y., and Thompson, R. F.,** Acute ethanol treatment modifies response properties and habituation of the DR-VR reflex in the isolated frog spinal cord, *Alcol. Clin. Exp. Res.,* 7, 194, 1983.
48. **Schmidt, R. F.,** Presynaptic inhibition in the vertebrate central nervous system, *Erg. Physiol.,* 63, 21, 1971.
49. **Spencer, P. S. and Schaumburg, H. N.,** Ultrastructural studies in the dying-back process. III. The evolution of experimental peripheral giant axonal degeneration, *J. Neuropathol. Exp. Neurol.,* 36, 276, 1977.
50. **Swanson, K. L. and Warnick, J. E.,** Tabun facilitates and depresses spinal reflexes in cat and neonatal rat spinal cords, *Soc. Neurosci. Abstr.,* 10, 417, 1984.
51. **Toennies, J. F.,** Reflex discharge from the spinal cord over the dorsal roots, *J. Neurophysiol.,* 1, 378, 1938.
52. **Toennies, J. F.,** Conditioning of afferent impulses by reflex discharge over the dorsal roots, *J. Neurophysiol.,* 2, 515, 1939.
53. **Willis, W. D. and Coggeshall, R. E.,** *Sensory Mechanisms of the Spinal Cord,* Plenum Press, New York, 1978.
54. **Yang, Q. Z. and Warnick, J. E.,** Effect of sarin and soman on spinal reflexes in the cat, *Soc. Neurosci. Abstr.,* 9, 285, 1983.
55. **Yang, Q. Z. and Warnick, N. E.,** Antagonism of organophosphate-induced depression of reflex activity in the neonatal rat spinal cord, *Soc. Neurosci. Abstr.,* 10, 417, 1984.
56. **Goldstein, B. D.,** Unpublished observation.

Chapter 7

PERIPHERAL NERVE CONDUCTION VELOCITIES AND EXCITABILITY

Rebecca J. Anderson

TABLE OF CONTENTS

I.   History of Conduction Velocity 52

II.   The Role of Geometry 52

III. The Role of Myelin 54

IV.   Measurement of Conduction Velocity 54
      A.   Clinical Measurements 54
      B.   Experimental Measurements 55

V.   The Effect of Neurotoxic Agents on Conduction Velocity 56
      A.   Types of Neurotoxic-Induced Changes 57
            1.   Conduction Block 57
            2.   Decreased Conduction Velocity 59
            3.   Increased Excitability 59
      B.   Remyelination 59
      C.   Agents which Affect Conduction Velocity 60

References 65

I. HISTORY OF CONDUCTION VELOCITY

Through the eighteenth and nineteenth centuries, a number of important and critical experimental observations were made which led to the first measurement of nerve conduction velocity. The details of these experiments have been reviewed.[1,2] The first critical observation was made by Galvani, who showed that frog muscles would twitch when electrically stimulated. This was largely thought to be a laboratory phenomenon since the source of electricity was man-made, a lead cell battery. Following Benjamin Franklin's now classic experiment with kite and key, which demonstrated that electricity was generated in the atmosphere, Galvani repeated his experiments. By hanging his frog preparation to a long wire during a storm, Galvani demonstrated that muscle could be stimulated by atmospheric as well as man-made electricity. With the invention of the galvanometer by Nobili, it was finally possible to measure naturally occurring currents, including those from biological tissues. Using this device, Matteucci demonstrated that when nerves and muscles are cut they emit an injury current which can be measured between the cut and intact sections of the muscle. Subsequently, du Bois-Raymond observed that nerves did not have to be injured in order to generate a current. When electrically stimulated, there was a change in the current generated by the nerves, a phenomenon he called the "negative variation". du Bois-Raymond suspected that this negative variation was an active process, traveling along the nerve, and was responsible for the muscle stimulation.

von Helmholtz devised the timing device which permitted the first measurement of conduction velocity of frog nerve. His experiment is illustrated in Figure 1. von Helmholtz electrically stimulated the end of a nerve (S1) at the same instant that a timing device was activated. The nerve activation resulted in a muscle twitch which mechanically stopped the same timing device. von Helmholtz then repeated the experiment after moving the stimulating electrodes closer to the muscle (S2). The time necessary to induce a muscle twitch (t2) was now shorter. By substrating the two times (t1 − t2), he determined the time necessary for the nerve impulse to travel the distance between the two stimulation sites (d). von Helmholtz calculated the conduction velocity of the nerve by dividing the distance traveled by the elapsed time.

II. THE ROLE OF GEOMETRY

There are a number of physical features of the nerve which determine the rate of impulse propagation. First, conduction velocity is directly proportional to axonal diameter. Rushton[3] calculated that, in peripheral nerves, conduction velocity increased by 6 m/sec for every micron added to the fiber diameter. Since the nerve axon does not remain constant over its entire length, conduction will decrease as the axon branches and fractionates into smaller-diameter components.

Branch points pose another problem for impulse propagation, since there is not only a change in diameter but also a quantal change in the surface area of the axon. This abrupt change seems to account for what has been called "branch point failure" of nerve conduction. The current density of an invading impulse may not be great enough for the action potential to be propagated down all branches simultaneously and conduction may thus proceed only along some or perhaps none of the branches.

Finally, the myelin sheath plays a critical role in the conduction velocity of larger-diameter fibers. Myelin is characterized by high electrical resistance and low capacitance, which permit it to function essentially as an electrical insulator. The sheath is discontinuous, with nodes of Ranvier at intervals approximately 1 μm apart along the axon. Impulse conduction is increased by the myelin since the impulse jumps in a saltatory manner from node to node. Not only can conduction proceed faster but it also consumes less energy than in nonmyelinated axons.[4]

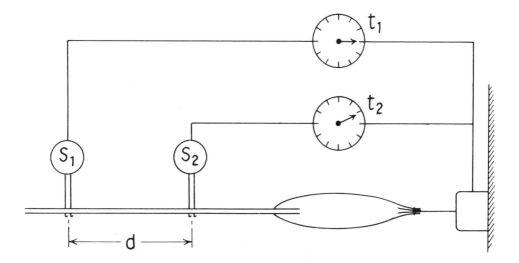

FIGURE 1. von Helmholtz method for calculating conduction velocity in frog nerve muscle preparation. Stimulation of the nerve at S_1 also started the timing of a clock. The subsequent muscle twitch activated a device which stopped the same clock. Stimulation at S_2 resulted in a shorter time for muscle contraction. The difference in time $(t_1 - t_2)$ represented the time required for the nerve action potential to travel between the two stimulation sites. By dividing this time by the distance between the electrodes (d), the first measure of nerve conduction velocity was obtained.

The physical and bioenergetic constraints of the axon-myelin relationship which determine conduction velocity and action potential propagation have recently been examined.[5] In myelinated nerves the geometry of the axon is such that the ratio of axon diameter to fiber diameter and of internodal length to fiber diameter are within the ranges which are most efficient for electrical conduction.[6] Thus, any alteration of the myelin will have an adverse effect on conduction. Although internodal distance and fiber diameters are matched to maximize conduction, the Schwann cells of peripheral nerves have a limit in the internodal lengths they are capable of generating, with 200 μm being the smallest. With this physiological limit, the smallest-diameter axon capable of efficient conduction is a diameter of about 1 μm. Thus, for peripheral nerves 1 μm becomes a critical diameter, above which myelin increases conduction and below which conduction is actually faster without myelin.[3]

The rule is somewhat different in the central nervous system (CNS), where axons are myelinated by glia. Central internodal distance can be as short as 10 μm. This means that central axons have a critical diameter of 0.2 μm, above which myelin increases conduction and below which myelination would be expected to decrease conduction. Electron microscopic studies have demonstrated myelinated axons as small as 0.2 μm in diameter, which is consistent with this view of nerve geometry relationships.[5]

Recent evidence by Funch and Faber[7] indicate that the electrophysiological parameters of the internodal axolemma and its sheath, and the type of cable structure used to represent a myelinated axon, need to be reconsidered. Experimental measurements indicated that the thickness of the myelin sheath is not the only determinant of conduction. Since the internodal axolemma itself appears to be an important barrier to transmembrane current, whereas the radial current flowing through the myelin may be relatively insignificant, altering myelin thickness would be expected to have only minimal effects on the action currents flowing in an axon. These observations are potentially very important when interpreting the effects of neurotoxic agents on conduction, since a number of peripheral neurotoxicants affect the myelin sheath.

III. THE ROLE OF MYELIN

Loss of myelin is the single most important factor in changing conduction velocity. Since impulse propagation in a demyelinated fiber is transformed from saltatory to continuous conduction, the speed of conduction can be markedly slowed.

In addition to the decreased speed of conduction, there is also a loss of efficiency in impulse propagation. This is the result of adaptive changes in myelinated axons which have shifted the distribution of ion channels for maximal utility during saltatory conduction. Rogart and Ritchie[8] have shown that the density of sodium channels at the nodes (about 10,000 per square micron) is much higher than under the myelin (less than 25 per square micron). This change apparently occurs during development since both sodium and potassium contribute to the action potential before myelination.[9] After the mature axon has been myelinated, the contribution of potassium to the action potential is attenuated. Thus, the uncovering of the high density of potassium channels during demyelination will tend to retard conduction by clamping the membrane at its resting potential.

Despite its well-known insulating properties and the role it plays in increasing conduction by creating saltatory impulse propagation, the myelin sheath has been recently shown not to limit transmembrane current flow.[7] Recordings obtained from within the myelin sheath of goldfish Mauthner axons showed that the apparent myelin resistance to current generated by action potentials is similar in magnitude to that of the internodal axolemma. This suggests that the sheath does not appreciably limit transmembrane current flow, presumably because there is a longitudinal shunt under the myelin and through the paranodal region. In some demyelinating diseases and other axonopathies, the safety factor for impulse conduction may be lowered by a loosening or reduction in the number of paranodal axoglial junctions.[7] Thus, the number or the tightness of the paranodal axoglial junctions may also be critical in determining the safety factor for impulse propagation.

Despite the marked change in conduction resulting from demyelination, it now seems increasingly evident that a combination of axonal degeneration and segmental demyelination is found in most neuropathies.[10] There is a close functional relationship between axons and Schwann cells. For example, the axon instructs the Schwann cells to produce myelin and conversely Schwann cells provide metabolic support for the axons.[10] Therefore, a neuropathic agent (even though it might initially attack only one component of the peripheral nerve) will ultimately affect the function of the other and conduction will be affected accordingly.

IV. MEASUREMENT OF CONDUCTION VELOCITY

Conduction velocity is the speed with which a nerve action potential travels along the nerve axon and is calculated in meters per second. A number of techniques have been employed to measure nerve conduction, both clinically and experimentally. Although the measurement is widely used, accurate measurements are difficult, due to a number of (usually) uncontrolled variables. The techniques employed and some of their limitations are explained below.

A. Clinical Measurements

The first clinical report of motor nerve conduction velocity was published in 1948.[11] The technique used clinically is largely unchanged from that used initially by von Helmholtz. Cutaneous stimulating electrodes are placed over a peripheral nerve (usually the median, peroneal, radial, or tibial) and the muscle action potential is recorded from electrodes placed over or in the muscle. Using two stimulation points along the nerve, the conduction velocity can be calculated. When measured in this way only the conduction velocity of the fastest fibers in the nerve bundle can be accurately recorded.

Sensory nerve conduction velocity is more difficult to record clinically. Many sensory axons are very small in diameter, have high thresholds, and cause discomfort to the patient when they are stimulated. Needle recording electrodes are inserted close to the nerve of interest (usually the sural, a pure cutaneous sensory nerve), and the nerve is stimulated distally near the foot.

Temperature and age have long been known to vary conduction velocity but it has only recently been reported that sex and the height of the patient also contribute to the normal variation in conduction velocity.[12] Despite correction for these factors, the normal variation between patients and the limited accuracy with which clinical measurements can be made both contribute to the difficulty in making an early diagnosis of peripheral neuropathy based upon conduction velocity changes.

Two recent developments have allowed clinical investigators to increase the information which can be obtained from clinical measures of conduction velocity. One is to take advantage of signal averaging techniques which resolve the very small, long latency, and slowly conducting components of the peripheral nerve compound action potential. Tackmann and Minkenberg[13] have used this technique to record from the median and sural nerves of normal and diseased patients. They demonstrated that, unlike the maximum conduction velocty, the slow components do not vary with age.

The other technique is one which uses computer iterative programming techniques to estimate the distribution of conduction velocities among the fibers in the nerve bundle. The characteristics of the single fiber action potential are used as the reference in this technique. The clinically recorded nerve compound action potential is then taken and "deconvoluted" by the computer into its individual components based on the single fiber example. The resulting information is a description of the distribution of fibers making up the nerve bundle, separated on the basis of their conduction velocities.[14,15] Using these techniques, information about the various components of the nerve can be distinguished and their relative susceptibility to neurotoxic agents can be determined.

B. Experimental Measurements

For a number of neurotoxicity studies, the nerve compound action potential has been recorded in animals using the same techniques as those used clinically. Noninvasive or *in situ* techniques have the advantage of permitting repeated measures in the same animal over time. Studies of the time course of the neurotoxicity and recovery can thus be followed in individual animals. In addition to peripheral nerves of the limbs, the rat tail nerve has also been widely used in neurotoxicology.[16] By placement of the recording electrodes distally or proximally, measures of motor or sensory nerve conduction, respectively, have been possible. Despite the advantages of following a single animal over extended periods, this technique suffers from the same disadvantages as clinical studies. Measurements are usually limited to the fastest components of the nerve and thus give only limited information about other components of the nerve.

More accurate measures of conduction velocity can be obtained from animals if the nerve is dissected and placed directly on stimulating and recording electrodes. Since the nerve lies in a straight line between the electrodes, accurate measurement of distance can be obtained. However, since most nerves are mixed and contain both sensory and motor fibers, the placement of stimulating and recording electrodes always results in antidromic conduction of some of the fibers.

The most useful information from measurements of conduction velocity have come from studies of single axons. If a representative sample of fibers in the nerve bundle (100 or more) is taken, the distribution of axons, based upon their individual conduction velocities, can be compared before and after exposure to neurotoxic substances. If the fibers are dissected from the ventral roots in the spinal cord, only motor axons will be included in the distribution.

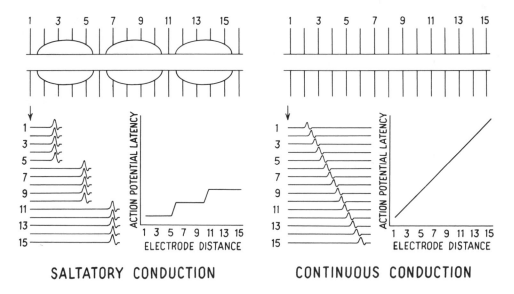

SALTATORY CONDUCTION   CONTINUOUS CONDUCTION

FIGURE 2.   Measurement of conduction along single nerve axons. The left panel shows the action potentials recorded at closely spaced sites along a single myelinated axon. The latency only changes as the recording site crosses a node of Ranvier. Plotting latency as a function of distance along the axon results in a step function. The right panel shows the recordings from an unmyelinated axon. In this case conduction is continuous and a plot of the data shows that latency is directly proportional to the distance along the axon.

If the fibers are dissected from the dorsal roots, only sensory axons will be included. Calculating conduction velocity from single axons is a tedious process and is somewhat biased in that the faster (larger-diameter) axons tend to be preferentially selected and are thus overrepresented. In addition, even in single-fiber studies, the measurement of conduction velocity is averaged over the length of the axon. In fact, conduction velocity of an axon changes over its course and depends on the changing axonal diameter, terminal branching, and degree of myelination.

Dissected single axons from rat have been used to demonstrate the changing conduction along its course.[17-19] This technique is illustrated in Figure 2. Using closely spaced recording electrodes at many intervals along the axon, the conduction can be recorded as the action potential crosses each node of Ranvier and exhibits a saltatory, discontinuous conduction in myelinated nerves. In unmyelinated axons (or the demyelinated regions of myelinated axon) continuous conduction is observed along the length of the axon. This technique is the most accurate representation of peripheral nerve conduction yet devised for monitoring the effects of neurotoxic agents. Its value is most applicable to studies in which effects on the myelin sheath are suspected.

V. THE EFFECT OF NEUROTOXIC AGENTS ON CONDUCTION VELOCITY

One way to assess neurotoxicity is on the basis of changes in nerve conduction. Depending on the type of neurotoxic substance, this can be a rather early indicator of peripheral nerve damage. However, in some cases, conduction velocity changes stay within the normal range even long after other signs of functional deficits are quite evident. It has even been argued[5] that optimal conduction is not always necessary for physiologic function, i.e., there is some allowance built into many nervous system functions so that alterations in conduction can occur without adverse effects on the organism. For example, although it is well known that conduction velocity is temperature dependent, the fluctuation in temperature (of several degrees) resulting from circadian rhythms does not disrupt most physiological functions.

It should be remembered that electrophysiological changes in conduction velocity reflect an inability of the nerve to carry impulses correctly. In a few cases of neurotoxins, such as tetradotoxin, there is a direct interruption of the sodium channel which is necessary for membrane depolarization. This has a devastating effect on impulse propagation. However, most other neuropathic agents which alter conduction velocity do so indirectly. In these cases it is only after the myelin sheath is disrupted or there are pathological changes in the cytoarchitecture or there are marked changes in the metabolism or active transport processes that a resultant change in conduction velocity is also evident. These conditions will eventually have an adverse effect on conduction velocity, but it is easy to understand that conduction velocity changes indicate a consequence and not a cause of most peripheral neurotoxicities.

Several careful studies comparing the effects on conduction velocity with the histopathological deficits suggest that the correlation is less than impressive. Behse and Buchthal,[20] in a clinical study, found that two thirds of the patients with normal electrophysiological activity in the sural nerve showed mild loss of fibers or signs of remyelination, indicating that quantitative histology was a more sensitive indicator of neurotoxicity than electrophysiological measurements. Similarly, Maxwell and LeQuesne[21] showed that the histopathology following hexachlorophene demyelination was more representative of the neurotoxicity than the measurement of conduction velocity.

In addition to these observations, the magnitude and length of exposure of the same agent may determine which of several neurotoxic actions may occur. It is now generally appreciated that an acute neuropathy produces an insult which is characterized by axonal degeneration and little segmental demyelination.[10] Conversely, if the neuropathy follows a more chronic course, conditions favor the development of demyelination and the likelihood of remyelinated (recovering) nerve fibers.[10]

A. Types of Neurotoxic-Induced Changes

Neurotoxic agents have been reported to produce several effects on nerve impulse conduction, including improving impulse transmission, decreasing conduction velocity, and producing complete conduction block. Table 1 lists examples taken from Thomas[10] and Bergmans[22] showing a number of conditions in which conduction velocity can be affected.

1. Conduction Block

Conduction block means failure of impulse propagation. This may be due to necrosis, of course, as in the case of Wallarian degeneration in which the axon has been lost altogether. However, conduction block need not depend on histopathologic changes. For instance, the pharmacologic basis of local anesthetics is to produce a reversible conduction block by preventing sodium conductance. If this is a permanent effect, such as with tetradotoxin, the consequences can be devastating for the animal. This type of irreversible conduction failure, which is quite common with many naturally occurring nerve toxins, leads to paralysis and rapid death of the organism. In less severe cases, conduction failure can result from membrane demyelination. After an acute demyelination the denuded axonal membrane exposes a strip of membrane in which the density of sodium channels is too low to support impulse conduction and is therefore electrically inexcitable. In addition, the presence of potassium channels in this area tend to clamp the demyelinated axon membrane close to the resting potential and thus further prevent conduction.[4]

It has been proposed that after demyelination there is a redistribution of sodium channels in an effort to restore impulse transmission.[6] However, despite this, the abrupt increase in surface area of excitable tissue at the demyelinated site may introduce an impedance mismatching and a resultant reduction in current density.[6] Morphological evidence has been presented[23] to demonstrate that after demyelination each of two possible changes in the nerve are possible: (1) there can be a concentration of ion channels in patches along the demyelinated

Table 1
**CONDITIONS AND AGENTS WHICH
PRODUCE VARYING DEGREES OF
CONDUCTION VELOCITY CHANGES**

I. Marked slowing in conduction velocity
   Diphtheritic neuropathy
   Experimental allergic neuroitis
   Lead poisoning
   Late phase hexachlorophene neuropathy
   Pressure neuropathy
   Murine muscular dystrophy
   Guillain-Barre syndrome
   Diabetic neuropathy
   Hereditary hypertrophic neuropathy
   Metachromatic leukodystrophy
II. Slight reduction in conduction velocity
   Iminodiproprionitrile neuropathy
   Distal to nerve compression
   Genetic- or streptozotocin-induced diabetic neuropathy
III. No selective reduction in conduction velocity
   Wallerian degeneration
   Alcoholic and porphyric neuropathy
   Thalidomide
   Isoniazid
   Thallium
   Triorthocresyl phosphate

axon which might contribute to conduction failure or, alternatively, (2) there can be relatively continuous distribution of channels along the axon which pemits continuous, rather than saltatory conduction along that part of the axon. Because of the reduced current density in th demyelinated region, there is significant capacitative and resistive shunting of the axonal current. If the adjacent section of membrane does not reach threshold, conduction failure results.[4]

The conduction failure, moreover, can be frequency dependent with low-frequency trains conducting normally but high-frequency trains failing.[4] Experimentally this phenomenon can be identified as a lengthening of the relative refractory period, and has been reported as an early sign of demyelination (i.e., prior to changes in conduction velocity) with two agents: lysophosphatidyl choline[24] and phenol.[25] Demyelinated axons are highly sensitive to temperature, with impulse conduction failing more frequently as temperature increases. This has been noted experimentally[4] and also is a well-known aspect of multiple sclerosis (MS), a demyelinating disease.[4]

Two recent lines of evidence point to the transition region between the myelinated and newly demyelinated segments as being particularly critical in determining whether conduction will fail. Using computer modeling techniques, Waxman and Wood[26] have presented simulations which show that ionic channel densities and distributions are most important in the transition region. By redistribution of channels in this region the impedance mismatch can be overcome and conduction restored through the remaining demyelinated region. The computer simulations indicated that conduction properties could be restored by redistribution of ion channels in a small band extending 100 μm from the site at which demyelination begins.

Secondly, Funch and Faber,[7] using microelectrode recordings of Mauthner axons, showed that there is a longitudinal shunt under the myelin and through the paranodal region of the axon. Therefore, any condition which would loosen or further reduce the number of paranodal axoglial junctions (which seem to regulate current flow), such as demyelination or some axonopathies, would be expected to lower the safety factor for impulse conduction. The data suggest that even minor changes in the paranodal axoglial junctions may have major consequences on impulse conduction.

2. Decreased Conduction Velocity

Short of conduction block, impulses can be slowed. This is most commonly the result of partial demyelination. If only some shunting of current takes place, it takes longer for the demyelinated region to reach threshold[4] but conduction may very well remain saltatory.[22] Alternatively, there may be a redistribution of sodium channels in the demyelinated region as a homeostatic mechanism to maintain conduction, which may result in a slowed rate which is continuous rather than saltatory.[22] Redistribution of existing channels, rather than introduction of new ionic channels, may be sufficient to support continuous impulse conduction in the demyelinated region.[6] Finally, there may be slowing of conduction in a peripheral nerve due to differential pathologic involvement of various fibers within the nerve bundle. If the fast-conducting fibers are most vulnerable, then conduction will appear to be slowed, despite normal transmission in the smaller-diameter, slower-conducting fibers.[4]

3. Increased Excitability

In some instances, demyelination can result in another phenomenon, i.e., increased excitability. If the axons remain intact, there is increased contact between neighboring axons which have been deprived of their insulating myelin sheaths. The consequence of this electrophysiologically is a "short circuiting" of the impulse traffic ephaptically across the two axons making contact. Ectopic excitability may also be generated in demyelinated axons, which could result in a tendency of the fibers to fire repetitively in response to a single stimulus. Evidence for both of these phenomenon have recently been reported in experimental cases of demyelination.[27,28]

Trains of impulses in partially demyelinated axons can be enhanced by mechanical stimulation of the lesioned area[27] or by maneuvers which lower the threshold for excitation such as lowering pCO_2 or serum calcium.[28] One contributing factor in this process seems to be the erratic distribution of potassium and sodium channels which follows demyelination. Rasminsky[28] has speculated that ion channel redistribution, local increases in axonal resistance, or changes in the extracellular concentration of potassium or calcium (from the activity of neighboring fibers) could all contribute to the increased activity of demyelinated fibers.

B. Remyelination

One complicating factor in interpretation of the electrophysiological responses is that remyelination may be occurring simultaneously with demyelination. It is therefore difficult to determine from a single measurement in a lesioned nerve whether the nerve is in the process of demyelination (and therefore getting worse) or in the process of remyelination (and therefore getting better). Only a sequence of measurements over a period of days or weeks can determine with certainty which process is dominant. The remyelination process results in a myelin sheath which ultimately will be thinner than the original and exhibit shorter internodal distances.[29] Therefore, some of the new nodes must necessarily have been formed at previous internodal sites. This means that considerable redistribution of ion channels and axonal functions must take place during the recovery from a demyelination incident. Despite these obvious differences, conduction velocities may approach normal values after remyelination. The only deficit appears to be a reduction in the amplitude of the nerve compound action potential, suggesting that some of the axons become necrotic and were lost entirely from the bundle.[30] However, those axons which remain are capable of restoring their former conduction velocity which means that the nerve axons can adapt to the new myelin in ways which improve impulse conduction. Waxman[6] has suggested a number of factors which promote conduction through remyelinated fibers, including reductions in internode distance, interposition of a larger excitable node proximal to the demyelinated region, a higher than normal density of sodium channels in the nodes proximal to the demyelinated area, and decreased axonal diameter in the demyelinated region.

C. Agents which Affect Conduction Velocity

Table 2 lists a number of recent studies which have reported neurotoxic agents which affect conduction velocity. Although this list is not meant to be exhaustive, it does point out the variability with which conduction velocity changes occur following exposure to toxic substances. As stated previously, changes in conduction velocity usually indicate the consequences of some other action of the toxic agent. Therefore, as more is learned about the histological, biochemical, and subcellular toxicities of various neuropathic substances, it becomes easier to explain the presence or absence of conduction velocity changes.

For instance, marked decreases in conduction velocity occur following exposure to hexachlorophene,[21,31] phenylmercuric acetate,[32] and lysophosphatidylcholine,[30] all of which are selective demyelinating agents. Demyelination also appears to be the reason for lead-induced reductions in conduction velocity in experimental studies.[33,34] However, lead-induced demyelination has not been reported in humans.[35] Despite this, there is nevertheless a marked slowing in conduction, especially of the slower-conducting fibers following lead exposure in patients,[36] occurring prior to other clinical neurological symptoms. Although there is considerable controversy among various clinical investigators, in patients which have been monitored over an extended period there appears to be a correlation between lead exposure (length and concentration factors) and nerve conduction velocity changes.[37]

IDPN and 2,5-hexanedione alter microtubule-neurofilament interactions.[38] This results in a selective stoppage of slow axonal transport, ballooning the proximal part of the axon and shrinkage of the distal axon.[39] The increased axonal diameter at periodic intervals along the axon decreases the charge density of an invading impulse, making it more difficult for the adjacent sections of membrane to reach threshold. Conduction, therefore, is slowed and may be blocked. In these cases, slowed conduction velocity reflects intracellular pathology, rather than demyelination.

A large body of data now exists regarding hexacarbon neurotoxicity.[94-108] The particular toxicity of hexane, as opposed to the hydrocarbons, appears to be the result of active metabolites, predominately 2,5-hexanedione. Multiple axonal swellings along the axon probably account for the early and marked reduction in conduction velocity, as impulse propagation is slowed at these sites. Demyelination at the swellings also contributes to the reduction in the individual conduction velocities of the axons in the nerve bundle following hexane exposure.[35]

Acrylamide, on the other hand, seems to reduce retrograde transport. Retention of rapidly transported proteins in the preterminal axons[39] is consistent with many other reports suggesting that acrylamide selectively disrupts nerve terminal function and only secondarily affects proximal segments of the axon.[40] This also explains the observations that axonal conduction velocity remains normal in animals with obvious behavioral deficits such as motor incoordination[41] and hindlimb weakness.[42]

The mild decreases in conduction velocity following acrylamide[43] appear to be due to a selective loss of the faster conducting axons. Rather than severe decreases in impulse conduction, acrylamide produces a marked decrease in the amplitude of the action potential which is the result of axonal damage.[35] Similar selective reductions in amplitude rather than in conduction velocity occur with zinc pyridinethione[44] and methyl mercury chloride[45] which also produce axonopathies, the latter by a selective effect on sensory axons.[46]

The reductions in conduction velocity following clioquinol exposure are restricted to the dorsal spinal roots and ascending tracts.[19] This agent produces a rather selective pathology

Table 2
STUDIES IN WHICH THE EFFECTS OF NEUROTOXIC AGENTS ON CONDUCTION VELOCITY HAVE BEEN MEASURED

Agent	Dose[a]	Species	Nerve	Effect No change	Effect Decrease	Ref.
Mercury (elemental)	Unintentional	Man	Median		X	49
			Peroneal	X		
			Ulnar	X		
Mercury (elemental)	Unintentional	Man	Superficial peroneal		X	50
			Ulnar	X		
			Median	X		
			Sural	X		
Mercury (elemental)	Unintentional	Man	Ulnar		X	51
Mercury (elemental/organic/inorganic)	Unintentional	Man	Ulnar	X		52
			Median	X		
Mercury (elemental/organic/inorganic	Unintentional	Man	Ulnar		X	53
			Median		X	
Methylmercury	Unintentional	Man	Median	X		54
			Peroneal	X		
			Tibial	X		
Methylmercury	Unintentional	Man	Median	X		55
Methylmercury	Unintentional	Man	Median	X		56
			Peroneal	X		
			Tibial	X		
Methylmercury	Unintentional	Man	Median	X		57
			Common peroneal	X		
			Posterior tibial	X		
Methylmercury	Unintentional	Man	Median	X		58
			Peroneal	X		
Methylmercury	5 mg/kg; 80 mg/kg	Rat	Sural	X		59
	5 mg/kg; 135 mg/kg	Rat	Sural		X	
	5 mg/kg; 35 mg/kg	Monkey	Median	X		
			Posterior tibial	X		
			Sural	X		
Methylmercury	0.5 mg; 22 mg	Rat	Tail		X	60
Methylmercury	10 mg/kg; 70 mg/kg	Rat	Sciatic		X	46
	2 mg/kg; 40 mg/kg	Rat				
Methylmercury	0.5 mg; 21 mg	Rat	Sciatic		X	45
			Tail		X	
Methylmercury	1 mg	Guinea pig	Sympathetic ganglion	X		61
Methoxy-ethylmercury	6 mg/kg; 420 mg/kg	Rabbit	Sciatic		X	62
Ethylmercury	Unintentional	Man	Median		X	63
			Ulnar		X	
			Peroneal		X	
Phenylmercury acetate	15 mg/kg; 1050 mg/kg	Rat	Sciatic		X	32
Lead (metallic/lead oxide)	Unintentional	Man	Ulnar		X	64
			Median		X	
Lead	Unintentional	Man	Median		X	65
			Peroneal	X		
			Sural	X		
Lead	Unintentional	Man	Median		X	66
Lead	Unintentional	Man	Peroneal	X		67
Lead	Unintentional	Man	Anterior tibial		X	68
Lead	Unintentional	Man	Peroneal		X	69

Table 2 (continued)
STUDIES IN WHICH THE EFFECTS OF NEUROTOXIC AGENTS ON CONDUCTION VELOCITY HAVE BEEN MEASURED

Agent	Dose[a]	Species	Nerve	No change	Decrease	Ref.
Lead	Unintentional	Man	Median		X	70
			Peroneal		X	
			Sural		X	
Lead	Unintentional	Man	Median		X	71
			Posterior tibial		X	
Lead	Unintentional	Man	Median	X	X	72
			Peroneal	X		
			Sural			
Lead	Unintentional	Man	Ulnar	X		73
			Peroneal	X		
			Sural	X		
Lead	Unintentional	Man	Radial		X	74
Lead	Unintentional	Man	Ulnar		X	75
			Median		X	
			Radial		X	
			Peroneal		X	
Lead	Unintentional	Man	Median		X	76
Lead	Unintentional	Man	Not specified	X		77
Lead	Unintentional	Man	Peroneal		X	78
Lead	Unintentional	Man	Median		X	79
			Ulnar		X	
			Deep peroneal		X	
			Posteior tibial		X	
Lead	Unintentional	Man	Median		X	80
			Ulnar		X	
			Peroneal		X	
			Radial		X	
Lead	Unintentional	Man	Radial	X		81
Lead	Unintentional	Man	Ulnar	X		82
Lead	Unintentional	Man	Ulnar		X	83
			Peroneal	X		
			Sural	X		
Lead	Unintentional	Man	Median		X	84
			Ulnar		X	
Lead	Unintentional	Man	Median		X	85
			Peroneal	X		
			Sural		X	
Lead acetate	30 µg/kg; 1.5 mg/kg	Man	Ulnar	X		86
Lead acetate	0.2% in drinking water	Rabbit	Sciatic		X	87
Lead acetate	0.1% in drinking water	Rabbit	Sciatic		X	88
Lead acetate	1 g/kg; 0.5 g/kg	Guinea pig	Sciatic		X	33
Lead carbonate	4% in food	Rat	Tail		X	34
Lead carbonate	50 mg/kg; 135 mg/kg	Monkey	Median	X		89
			Anterior tibial	X		
Zinc acetate	0.2% in drinking water	Rabbit	Sciatic	X		87
Zinc pyrithione	250 ppm in food	Rat	Sural	X		90
			Sciatic	X		
Zinc pyrithione	250 ppm in food	Rat	Sural	X		44
Arsenic trioxide	Unintentional	Man	Ulnar	X		91
			Sural	X		
			Common peroneal	X		
Hydrocarbon mixture	Unintentional	Man	Median		X	92
			Peroneal		X	

Table 2 (continued)
STUDIES IN WHICH THE EFFECTS OF NEUROTOXIC AGENTS ON
CONDUCTION VELOCITY HAVE BEEN MEASURED

Agent	Dose[a]	Species	Nerve	No change	Decrease	Ref.
Organic solvents	Unintentional	Man	Median		X	93
			Peroneal		X	
			Ulnar	X		
n-Hexane	Unintentional	Man	Peroneal		X	94
			Median		X	
			Ulnar		X	
n-Hexane	Unintentional	Man	Median		X	95
			Ulnar		X	
			Peroneal		X	
			Tibial		X	
n-Hexane	Unintentional	Man	Median		X	96
			Ulnar		X	
			Peroneal		X	
			Tibial		X	
n-Hexane	Unintentional	Man	Ulnar		X	97
			Median		X	
			Peroneal		X	
n-Hexane	3000 ppm inhaled	Rat	Tail		X	98
n-Hexane	1000 ppm inhaled	Rat	Tail		X	99
n-Hexane	0.4—1.2 ml/day;36.4 ml	Rat	Tail		X	100
n-Hexane	3000 ppm inhaled	Rat	Tail		X	101
n-Hexane	500—1500 ppm inhaled	Rat	Tail		X	102
n-Hexane	325 mg/kg; 10.6 g/day	Rat	Tail		X	103
2,5-Hexanedione	200—300 mg/kg; 10.5 g/kg	Rat	Tail		X	104
2,5-Hexanedione	400 mg/kg; 8 g/kg	Rat	Tail		X	105
	200 mg/kg; 14 g/kg	Rat	Tail		X	
2,5-Hexanedione	485 mg/kg; 1.9 g/kg	Rat	Tail		X	103
2,5-Hexanedione	0.1—0.5% in drinking water	Rat	Sciatic		X	106
2,5-Hexanedione	0.1 mg/kg; 29.4 mg/kg	Baboon	Tibial			48
			Median			100
			Sural		X	
2-Methylpentane	0.4—1.2 ml/day; 36.4 ml	Rat	Tail			
3-Methylpentane	0.4—1.2 ml/day; 36.4 ml	Rat	Tail		X	100
Methylcyclopentane	0.4—1.2 ml/day; 36.4 ml	Rat	Tail		X	100
2-Hexanol	400 mg/kg; 42 g/kg	Rat	Tail		X	107
2-Hexanol	101.2—151.8 mg/kg; 25 g/kg	Rat	Tail		X	108
1-Hexanol	102.5 mg/kg; 18.5 g/kg	Rat	Tail		X	108
n-Pentane	3000 ppm inhaled	Rat	Tail	X		98
n-Heptane	3000 ppm inhaled	Rat	Tail	X		98
n-Heptane	3000 ppm inhaled	Rat	Tail	X		98
2-Octanol	400 mg/kg; 42 g/kg	Rat	Tail	X		107
Toluene	1000 ppm inhaled	Rat	Tail	X		109
Hexachlorophene	1000 ppm in food	Rat	Sural		X	44
Hexachlorophene	25—70 mg/kg	Rat	Sciatic		X	31
Hexachlorophene	800—1000 ppm in food	Rat	Sciatic		X	21

Table 2 (continued)
STUDIES IN WHICH THE EFFECTS OF NEUROTOXIC AGENTS ON CONDUCTION VELOCITY HAVE BEEN MEASURED

Agent	Dose[a]	Species	Nerve	No change	Decrease	Ref.
Carbon diisulfide	700 ppm inhaled	Rat	Sciatic		X	110
Acrylamide	Unintentional	Man	Median	X		111
			Tibial	X		
Acrylamide	15 mg/kg; 1.5 g/kg	Baboon	Median		X	112
Acrylamide	10—15 mg/kg; 1.5 g/kg	Baboon	Median		X	43
			Anterior tibial		X	
Acrylamide	7 mg/kg	Dog	Sciatic		X	113
			Vagus		X	
Acrylamide	15 mg/kg; 1.7 g/kg	Cat	Posterior tibial		X	114
			Greater splanchnic		X	
Acrylamide	10 mg/kg; 920 mg/kg	Cat	Sciatic	X		115
Acrylamide	10 mg/kg; 670 mg/kg	Cat	Medial			116
			Gastrocnemius	X		
Acrylamide	10 mg/kg; 200 mg/kg	Cat	Medial			40
			Gastrocnemius	X		
Acrylamide	30 mg/kg; 150—300 mg/kg	Cat	Soleus	X		41
Acrylamide	7.5—30 mg/kg; 300 mg/kg	Cat	Soleus	X		117
Acrylamide	15 mg/kg; 150 mg/kg	Cat	Soleus	X		118
Acrylamide	15 mg/kg; 300 mg/kg	Rat	Cervical			119
			Sympathetic trunk	X		
Acrylamide	100 mg/kg; 900 mg/kg	Mouse	Sural		X	120
			Sciatic		X	
DFP	2 mg/kg	Cat	Soleus	X		121
DFP	2 mg/kg	Cat	Soleus	X		122
Lysophosphatidylcholine	4.5 μℓ of 1% solution	Rat	Posterior tibial		X	123
Polychlorinated biphenyls	Unintentional	Man	Not specified		X	124
Diphenyl	Unintentional	Man	Median	X		125
			Ulnar		X	
			Peroneal	X		
			Posterior tibial	X		
Clioquinol	200 mg/kg; 39.2 g/kg	Baboon	Tibial	X		48
			Median	X		
			Sural	X		
Clioquinol	600 mg/kg; 176.4 g/kg	Baboon	Tibial		X	48
			Median	X		
			Sural	X		
Vincristine	Unintentional	Man	Peroneal	X		126
			Median	X		
Isoniazid	150 mg/kg, 3 g/kg	Rat	Cervical Sympathetic Trunk	X		119
Ethanol	11—12 g/kg; 1.5 kg/kg	Rat	Tail	X		127

[a]   Single daily dose; total cumulative dose.

of the proximal sensory nerve endings and CNS axons,[47] which is consistent with a marked slowing in the somatosensory evoked potentials (SEPs) in baboons.[48]

In conclusion, one must be cautious in using conduction velocity in studies of neurotoxicity. Although conduction velocity changes almost always indicate neurotoxicity, the converse is not always true. Many neurotoxic agents, including some of those cited here, can cause considerable damage or disruption of nerve function without altering conduction velocity. Secondly, the speed of impulse propagation may not be as important to the organism as other features of propagation (for instance, transmission of high- and low-frequency impulses). Finally, since conduction velocity changes under normal physiological conditions (for instance, diurnally), some investigators have even questioned whether small changes in conduction velocity are meaningful. Therefore, the use of conduction velocity as a measure of neurotoxicity should be reserved as a confirmatory parameter which may correlate with other pathophysiological changes. However, it does not stand on its own as a hallmark of neurotoxicity.

REFERENCES

1. **Brazier, M. A. B.,** *Handbook of Physiology, Section I: Neurophysiology,* Vol. I, Field, J., Ed., American Physiological Society, Washington, D.C., 1959, 1.
2. **Schuetze, S. M.,** The discovery of the action potential, *Trends Neurosci.,* 6, 164, 1983.
3. **Rushton, W. A. H.,** *J. Physiol.,* 115, 101, 1951.
4. **Waxman, S. G.,** Membranes, myelin and the pathophysiology of multiple sclerosis, *N. Engl. J. Med.,* 306, 1529, 1982.
5. **Waxman, S. G.,** Action potential propagation and conduction velocity — new perspectives and questions, *Trends Neurosci.,* 6, 157, 1983.
6. **Waxman, S. G.,** Prerequisites for conduction in demyelinated fibers, *Neurology,* 28, 27, 1978.
7. **Funch, P. G. and Faber, D. S.,** Measurement of myelin sheath resistances: implications for axonal conduction and pathophysiology, *Science,* 225, 538, 1984.
8. **Rogart, R. B. and Ritchie, J. M.,** *Myelin,* Morell, P., Ed., Plenum Press, New York, 1977, 117.
9. **Waxman, S. G. and Foster, R. E.,** Ionic channel distribution and heterogeneity of the axon membrane in myelinated fibers, *Brain Res. Rev.,* 2, 205, 1980.
10. **Thomas, P. K.,** The morphological basis for alterations in nerve conduction in peripheral neuropathy, *Proc. R. Soc. Med.,* 64, 295, 1971.
11. **Hodes, R., Larrabee, M. G., and German, W.,** *Arch. Neurol. Psychiatr.,* 60, 340, 1948.
12. **Lang, A. H., Forsstrom, J., Bjorkqvist, S.-E., and Kuusela, V.,** Statistical variation of nerve conduction velocity. An analysis in normal subjects and uraemic patients, *J. Neurol. Sci.,* 33, 229, 1977.
13. **Tackmann, W. and Minkenberg, R.,** Nerve conduction velocity of small components in human sensory nerves — studies in normal and diseased nerves, *Eur. Neurol.,* 16, 270, 1977.
14. **Cummons, K. L., Dorfman, L. J., and Perkel, D. H.,** Nerve conduction velocity distributions: a method for estimation based upon two compound action potentials, in *Conduction Velocity Distributions: A Population Approach to Electrophysiology of Nerve,* Alan R. Liss, New York, 1981, 181.
15. **Sax, D. S., Kovacs, Z. L., Johnson, T. L., and Feldman, R. G.,** Clinical applications of the estimation of nerve conduction velocity distributions, *Prog. Clin. Biol. Res.,* 52, 113, 1981.
16. **Miyoshi, T. and Goto, I.,** Serial in vivo determinations of nerve conduction velocity in rat tails. Physicological and pathological changes, *EEG Clin. Neurophys.,* 35, 125, 1973.
17. **Rasminsky, M. and Sears, T. A.,** Internodal conduction in undissected demyelinated nerve fibers, *J. Physiol.,* 227, 323, 1977.
18. **Bostock, H. and Sears, T. A.,** The internodal axon membrane: electrical excitability and continuous conduction in segmental demyelination, *J. Physiol.,* 280, 273, 1978.
19. **Homma, S., Kotaki, H., Mizote, M., Nakajima, Y., and Tamura, Z.,** Saltatory conduction of peripheral nerve impulse in clioquinol treated rats, *Neurosci. Lett.,* 45, 259, 1984.
20. **Behse, F. and Buchthal, F.,** Sensory action potentials and biopsy of the sural nerve in neuropathy, *Brain,* 101, 473, 1978.
21. **Maxwell, I. C. and LeQuesne, P. M.,** Conduction velocity in hexachlorophene neuropathy: correlation between electrophysiological and histological findings, *J. Neurol. Sci.,* 43, 95, 1979.
22. **Bergmans, J. A.,** Neurophysiological features of experimental and human neuropathies, in *Clinical and Biological Aspects of Peripheral Nerve Diseases,* Alan R. Liss, New York, 1983, 73.
23. **Foster, R. E., Whalen, C. C., and Waxman, S. G.,** Reorganization of the axon membrane in demyelinated peripheral nerve fibers: morphological evidence, *Science,* 210, 661, 1980.
24. **Smith, K. J. and Hall, S. M.,** Nerve conduction during peripheral demyelination and remyelination, *J. Neurol. Sci.,* 48, 201, 1980.
25. **Anderson, R. J.,** Relative refractory period as a measure of peripheral nerve neurotoxicity, *Toxicol. Appl. Pharmacol.,* 71, 391, 1983.

26. **Waxman, S. G. and Wood, S. L.,** Impulse conduction in inhomogeneous axons: effects of variation in voltage-sensitive ionic conductances on invasion of demyelinated axon segments and preterminal fibers, *Brain Res.,* 294, 111, 1984.
27. **Smith, K. J. and McDonald, W. I.,** Spontaneous and mechanically evoked activity due to central demyelinating lesion, *Nature (London),* 286, 154, 1980.
28. **Rasminsky, M.,** Ectopic impulse generation in pathological nerve fibres, *Trends Pharmaceut. Sci.,* 6, 388, 1983.
29. **Gledhill, R. F., Harrison, B. M., and McDonald, W. I.,** Pattern of remyelination in the CNS, *Nature (London),* 244, 443, 1973.
30. **Smith, K. J., Blakemore, W. F., and McDonald, W. I.,** Central remyelination restores secure conduction, *Nature (London),* 280, 395, 1979.
31. **DeJesus, P. V. and Pleasure, D. E.,** Hexachlorophene neuropathy, *Arch. Neurol.,* 29, 180, 1973.
32. **Slizewski, M.,** Influence of chronic administration of phenylmercuric acetate on the peripheral nerve system of rat, *Neuropathol. Pol.,* 13, 471, 1975.
33. **Fullerton, P. M.,** Chronic peripheral neuropathy produced by lead poisoning in guinea pigs, *Neuropathol. Exp. Neurol.,* 25, 214, 1966.
34. **Ohnishi, A., Schilling, K., Brimijoin, W. S., Lambert, E. H., Fairbanks, V. F., and Dyck, P. J.,** Lead neuropathy. I. Morphometry, nerve conduction and choline acetyltransferase transport: new finding of endoneurial edema associated with segmental demyelination, *J. Neuropathol. Exp. Neurol.,* 36, 499, 1977.
35. **LeQuesne, P. M.,** Electrophysiological investigation of toxic neuropathies, *Acta Neurol. Scand.,* 66, 75, 1982.
36. **Seppalainen, A. M. and Hernberg, S.,** Sensitive technique for detecting subclinical lead neuropathy, *Br. J. Ind. Med.,* 29, 443, 1972.
37. **Seppalainen, A. M.,** Lead poisoning: neurophysiological aspects, *Acta Neurol. Scand.,* 66, 177, 1982.
38. **Griffin, J. W., Price, D. L., and Hoffman, P. N.,** Neurotoxic probes of the axonal cytoskeleton, *Trends Neurosci.* 6, 490, 1983.
39. **Jakobsen, J., Brimijoin, S., and Sidenius, P.,** Axonal transport in neuropathy, *Muscle Nerve,* 6, 164, 1983.
40. **Summer, A. J. and Asbury, A. K.,** Physiological studies of the dying-back phenomenon. Muscle stretch afferents in acrylamide neuropathy, *Brain,* 98, 91, 1975.
41. **Lowndes, H. E., Baker, T., Michelson, L. P., and Vincent-Ablazey, M.,** Attenuated dynamic responses of primary endings of muscle spindles: a basis for depressed tendon responses in acrylamide neuropathy, *Ann. Neurol.,* 3, 433, 1978.
42. **Tilson, H. A. and Cabe, P. A.,** The effects of acrylamide given acutely or in repeated doses on fore- and hind-limb function of rats, *Toxicol. Appl. Pharmacol.,* 47, 253, 1979.
43. **Hopkins, A. P. and Gilliatt, R. W.,** Motor and sensory conduction velocity in the baboon: normal values and changes during acrylamide neuropathy, *J. Neurol. Neurosurg. Psychiatry,* 34, 415, 1971.
44. **deJesus, C. P. V., Towfighi, J., and Snyder, D. R.,** Sural nerve conduction study in the rat: a new technique for studying experimental neuropathies, *Muscle Nerve,* 1, 162, 1978.
45. **Misumi, J.,** Electrophysiological studies in vivo on peripheral nerve function and their application to peripheral neuropathy produced by organic mercury in rats. III. Effects of methylmercuric chloride on compound action potentials in the sciatic and tail nerve in rats, *Kumamoto Med. J.,* 32, 15, 1979.
46. **Somjen, G. G., Herman, S. P., and Klein, R.,** Electrophysiology of methyl mercury poisoning, *J. Pharmacol. Exp. Ther.,* 186, 579, 1973.
47. **Krinke, G., Schaumburg, H. H., Spencer, P. S., Thomann, P., and Hess, R.,** Clioquinol and 2,5-hexanedione produce different types of distal axonopathy: a comparative experimental study in the dog, *Acta Neuropathol.,* 47, 213, 1979.
48. **Thomas, P. K., Bradley, D. J., Bradley, W. A., Degen, P. H., Krinke, G., Muddle, J., Schaumburg, H. H., Skelton-Stroud, P. N., Thomann, P., and Tzebelikos, E.,** Correlated nerve conduction, somatosensory evoked potential and neuropathological studies in clioquinol and 2,5-hexanedione neurotoxicity in the baboon, *J. Neurol. Sci.,* 64, 277, 1984.
49. **Albers, J. W., Cavender, G. D., Levine, S. P., and Langolf, G. D.,** Asymptomatic sensorimotor polyneuropathy in workers exposed, *Neurology,* 32, 1168, 1982.
50. **Iyer, K., Goodgold, J., Eberstein, A., and Berg, P.,** Mercury poisoning in a dentist, *Arch. Neurol.,* 33, 788, 1976.
51. **Levin, S. P., Cavender, G. D., Langolf, G. D., and Albers, J. W.,** Elementary mercury exposure: peripheral neurotoxicity, *Br. J. Ind. Med.,* 39, 136, 1982.
52. **Triebig, G., Schaller, K. H., and Valentin, H.,** Studies of neurotoxicity of chemical substances at the workplace. I. Determination of the motor and sensory nerve conduction velocity in persons occupationally exposed to mercury, *Int. Arch. Occup. Environ. Health,* 48, 119, 1981.

53. **Triebig, G. and Schaller, K. H.,** Neurotoxic effects in mercury-exposed workers, *Neurobehav. Toxicol. Teratol.,* 4, 717, 1982.
54. **Rustam, H., Von Burg, R., Amin-Zaki, L., and El Hassani, S.,** Evidence for a neuromuscular disorder in methylmercury poisoning, *Arch. Environ. Health,* 30, 190, 1975.
55. **Le Quesne, P. M., Damluji, S. F., and Rustam, H.,** Electrophysiological studies of peripheral nerves in patients with organic mercury poisoning, *J. Neurol. Neurosurg. Psych.,* 37, 333, 1974.
56. **Von Burg, R. and Rustam, H.,** Electrophysiological investigations of methylmercury intoxication in humans. Evaluation of peripheral nerve by conduction velocity and electromyography, *EEG Clin. Neurophysiol.,* 37, 381, 1974.
57. **Snyder, R. D. and Seelinger, D. F.,** Methylmercury poisoning. Clinical follow-up and sensory nerve conduction studies, *J. Neurol. Neurosurg. Psych.,* 39, 701, 1976.
58. **Von Burg, R. and Rustam, H.,** Conduction velocities in methylmercury poisoned patients, *Bull. Environ. Contam. Toxicol.,* 12, 1, 1974.
59. **Murai, Y., Shiraishi, S., Yamashita, Y., Ohnishi, A., and Arimura, K.,** Neurophysiological effects of methyl mercury on the nervous system, *EEG Clin. Neurophysiol.,* 36, 682, 1982.
60. **Misumi, J. and Nomura, S.,** An electrophysiological method for examination in vivo of peripheral neuropathy due to organic mercury poisoning in rats, *Proc. Int. Congr. Occup. Health,* 1, 239, 1980.
61. **Juang, M. S. and Yonemura, K.,** Increased spontaneous transmitter release from presynaptic nerve terminal by methylmercuric chloride, *Nature (London),* 256, 211, 1975.
62. **Lehotzky, K., Bordas, S., Sebok, J., and Batskor, I. A.,** Neurotoxic effect of methoxy-ethyl-mercury chloride, *Acta Med. Acad. Sci. Hung. Tomus.,* 28, 295, 1971.
63. **Cinca, I., Dumitrescu, I., Onaca, P., Serbanescu, A., and Nestorescu, B.,** Accidental ethyl mercury poisoning with nervous system, skeletal muscle, and myocardium injury, *J. Neurol. Neurosurg. Psych.,* 43, 143, 1979.
64. **Triebig, G., Weltle, D., and Valentin, H.,** Investigations on neurotoxicity of chemical substances at the workplace. V. Determination of the motor and sensory nerve conduction velocity in persons occupationally exposed to lead, *Int. Arch. Occup. Environ. Health,* 53, 189, 1984.
65. **Bordo, B., Massetto, N., Musicco, M., Filippini, G., and Boeri, R.,** Electrophysiologic changes in workers with ''low'' blood lead levels, *Am. J. Ind. Med.,* 3, 23, 1982.
66. **Seppalainen, A. M. and Hernberg, S.,** Subclinical lead neuropathy, *Am. J. Ind. Med.,* 1, 413, 1980.
67. **Landrigan, P. J., Baker, E. L., Feldman, R. G., Cox, D. H., Eden, K. V., Orenstein, W. A., Mather, J. A., Yankel, A. J., and Von Lindern, I. H.,** Increased lead absorption with anemia and slowed nerve conduction in children near a lead smelter, *J. Pediatr.,* 89, 904, 1976.
68. **Feldman, R. G., Haddow, J., Kopito, L., and Schwachman, H.,** Altered peripheral nerve conduction velocity. Chronic lead intoxication in children, *Am. J. Dis. Child.,* 125, 39, 1973.
69. **Behse, F., Pach, J., and Dorndorf, W.,** Polyneuropathy due to lead poisoning: clinical electrophysiological and bioptic findings, *Z. Neurol.,* 202, 209, 1972.
70. **Buchthal, F. and Behse, F.,** Electrophysiology and nerve biopsy in men exposed to lead, *Br. J. Ind. Med.,* 36, 135, 1979.
71. **Araki, S. and Honma, T.,** Relationships between lead absorption and peripheral nerve conduction velocities in lead workers, *Scand. J. Work Environ. Health,* 2, 225, 1976.
72. **Bordo, B. M., Filippini, G., Massetto, N., Musicco, M., and Boeri, R.,** Electrophysiological study of subjects occupationally exposed to lead and with low levels of lead poisoning, *Scand. J. Work Environ. Health,* 8, 142, 1982.
73. **Baloh, R. W., Spivey, G. H., Brown, C. P., Morgan, D., Campion, D. S., Browdy, B. L., Valentine, J. L., Gonick, H. C., Massey, F. J., and Culver, B. D.,** Subclinical effects of chronic increased lead absorption: a prospective study. II. Results of baseline neurologic testing, *J. Occup. Med.,* 21, 409, 1979.
74. **Lilis, R., Fischbein, A., Eisinger, J., Blumberg, W. E., Diamond, S., Anderson, H. A., Rom, W., Rice, C., Sarkozi, L., Kon, S., and Selikoff, I. J.,** Prevalence of lead disease among secondary lead smelter workers and biological indicators of lead exposure, *Environ. Res.,* 14, 255, 1977.
75. **Ashby, J. A.,** A neurological and biochemical study of early lead poisoning, *Br. J. Ind. Med.,* 37, 133, 1980.
76. **Araki, S., Honma, T., Yanagihara, S., and Ushio, K.,** Recovery of slowed nerve conduction velocity in lead-exposed workers, *Int. Arch. Occup. Environ. Health,* 46, 151, 1980.
77. **Sachs, K. H., McCaughran, D. A., Krall, V., Rozenfeld, I. H., and Yongsmith, N.,** Lead poisoning without encephalopathy. Effect of early diagnosis on neurologic and psychologic salvage, *Am. J. Dis. Child.,* 133, 786, 1979.
78. **Feldman, R. G., Hayes, M. K., Younes, R., and Aldrich, F. D.,** Lead neuropathy in adults and children, *Arch. Neurol.,* 34, 481, 1977.
79. **Seppalainen, A. M., Hernberg, S., Vesanto, R., and Kock, B.,** Early neurotoxic effects of occupational lead exposure: a prospective study, *Neurotoxicology,* 4, 181, 1983.

80. **Vasilescu, C.,** Motor nerve conduction velocity and electromyogram in chronic lead poisoning, *Rev. Roum. Neurol.,* 10, 221, 1973.

81. **Mostafa, M., El-Sewefy, A. Z., and Hamid, T. A.,** Clinical, biochemical, and electromyographic study in Egyptian lead workers, *Med. Lavoro,* 63, 109, 1972.

82. **Paulev, P. E., Gry, C., and Dossing, M.,** Motor nerve conduction velocity in asymptomatic lead workers, *Int. Arch. Occup. Environ. Health,* 7, 37, 1979.

83. **Spivey, G. H., Baloh, R. W., Brown, C. P., Browdy, B. L., Campion, D. S., Valentine, J. L., Morgan, D. E., and Culver, D. B.,** Subclinical effects of chronic increased lead absorption — a prospective study. III. Neurologic findings at follow-up examination, *J. Occup. Med.,* 22, 607, 1980.

84. **Seppalainen, A. M. and Hernberg, S.,** A follow-up study of nerve conduction velocities in lead exposed workers, *Neurobehav. Toxicol. Teratol.,* 4, 721, 1982.

85. **Singer, R., Valciukas, J. A., and Lilis, R.,** Lead exposure and nerve conduction velocity: the differential time course of sensory and motor nerve effects, *Neurotoxicology,* 4, 193, 1983.

86. **Verberk, M. M.,** Motor nerve conduction velocity in volunteers ingesting inorganic lead for 49 days, *Int. Arch. Occup. Environ. Health,* 39, 141, 1976.

87. **Hietanen, E., Kilpio, J., Loivusaari, U., Nevalainen, T., Narhi, M., Savolainen, H., and Vainio, H.,** Neurotoxicity of lead in rabbits, in *Mechanisms of Toxicity and Hazard Evaluation,* Holmstedt, B., Lauwerys, R., Mercier, M., and Roberfroid, M., Eds., Elsevier/North-Holland, Amsterdam, 1980, 67.

88. **Hietanen, E., Kilpio, J., Narhi, M., Savolainen, H., and Vainio, H.,** Biotransformational and neurophysiological changes in rabbits exposed to lead, *Arch. Environ. Contam. Toxicol.,* 9, 337, 1980.

89. **Hopkins, A.,** Experimental lead poisoning in the baboon, *Br. J. Ind. Med.,* 27, 130, 1970.

90. **Snyder, D. R., de Jesus, C. P. V., Towfighi, J., Jacoby, R. O., and Wedig, J. H.,** Neurological, microscopic, and enzymehistochemical assessment of zinc pyrithione toxicity, *Food Cosmet. Toxicol.,* 17, 651, 1979.

91. **Feldman, R. G., Niles, C. A., Kelly-Hayes, M., Sax, D. S., Dixon, W. J., Thompson, D. J., and Landau, E.,** Peripheral neuropathy in arsenic smelter workers, *Neurology,* 29, 939, 1979.

92. **Mutti, A., Cavatorta, A., Lommi, G., Lotta, S., and Franchini, I.,** Neurophysiological effects of long-term exposure to hydrocarbon mixtures, *Arch. Toxicol.,* 5, 120, 1982.

93. **Mutti, A., Cavatorta, A., Lucertini, S., Arfini, G., Falzoi, M., and Franchini, I.,** Neurophysiological changes in workers exposed to organic solvents in a shoe factory, *Scand. J. Work Environ. Health,* 8, 136, 1982.

94. **Bravaccio, F., Ammendola, A., Barruffo, L., and Cralomagno, S.,** H-reflex behavior in glue (n-hexane) neuropathy, *Clin. Toxicol.,* 18, 1369, 1981.

95. **Iida, M., Yamamura, Y., and Sobue, I.,** Electromyographic findings and conduction velocity on *n*-hexane polyneuropathy, *Electromyography,* 9, 247, 1969.

96. **Iida, M.,** Neurophysiological studies of n-hexane polyneuropathy in the sandal factory, *Electroencephalog. Clin. Neurophysiol.,* 36, 671, 1982.

97. **Mutti, A., Ferri, F., Lommi, G., Lotta, S., Lucertini, S., and Franchini, I.,** *n*-Hexane-induced changes in nerve conduction velocities and somatosensory evoked potentials, *Int. Arch. Occup. Environ. Health,* 51, 45, 1982.

98. **Takeuchi, Y., Ono, Y., Hisanaga, N., Kitoh, J., and Sugiura, Y.,** A comparative study of the toxicity of *n*-pentane, *n*-hexane, and *n*-heptane to the peripheral nerve of the rat, *Clin. Toxicol.,* 18, 1395, 1981.

99. **Rebert, C. S., Houghton, P. W., Howd, R. A.,and Pryor, G. T.,** Effects of hexane on the brainstem auditory response and caudal nerve action potential, *Neurobehav. Toxicol. Teratol.,* 4, 79, 1982.

100. **Ono, Y., Takeuchi, Y., and Hisanaga, N.,** A comparative study on the toxicity of n-hexane and its isomers on the peripheral nerve, *Int. Arch. Occup. Environ. Health,* 48, 289, 1981.

101. **Takeuchi, Y., Ono, Y., Hisanaga, N., Kitoh, J., and Sugiura, Y.,** A comparative study on the neurotoxcity of *n*-pentane, *n*-hexane, and *n*-heptane in the rat, *Br. J. Ind. Med.,* 37, 241, 1980.

102. **Rebert, C. S. and Sorenson, S. S.,** Concentration-related effects on evoked responses from brain and peripheral nerve of the rat, *Neurobehav. Toxicol. Teratol.,* 5, 69, 1983.

103. **Misumi, J., Kawakami, M., Hitoshi, T., and Nomura, S.,** Effects of *n*-hexane, methyl-*n*-butyl ketone and 2,5-hexanedione on the conduction velocity of motor and sensory nerve fibers in rats' tail, *Sangyo Igaku,* 21, 180, 1979.

104. **Nagano, M., Sato, K., Eto, K., Misumi, J., and Nomura, S.,** An experimental study on electrophysiological and histopathological changes in 2,5-hexanedione-intoxicated rats, *Sangyo Igaku,* 25, 77, 1983.

105. **Nagano, M., Misumi, J., Kaisaku, J., and Hitoshi, T.,** Experimental studies on peripheral neuropathy due to chemical substances: electrophysiological technique for detecting peripheral neuropathy and its application to 2,5 hexanedione rats, *Kyushu Yakugakkai Kaiho,* 36, 91, 1982.

106. **Nachtman, J. P. and Couri, D.,** Biophysical and electrophysiological studies of hexanedione neurotoxicity, *Neurotoxicology,* 2, 541, 1981.

107. **Musumi, J., Nagano, M., and Nomura, S.,** An experimental study on the neurotoxicity of 2-octanone and 2-hexanol, a metabolite of *n*-hexane, *Sangyo Igaku,* 24, 475, 1982.

108. **Perbellini, L., DeGrandis, D., Semenzato, F., Rizzuto, N., and Simonati, A.,** An experimental study on the neurotoxicity of n-hexane metabolites hexanol-1 and hexanol-2, *Toxicol. Appl. Pharmacol.,* 46, 421, 1978.

109. **Takeuchi, Y., Ono, Y., and Hisanaga, N.,** An experimental study on the combined effects of *n*-hexane and toluene on the peripheral nerve of the rat, *Br. J. Ind. Med.,* 38, 14, 1981.

110. **Colombi, A., Maroni, M., Picchi, O., Rota, E., Castano, P., and Foa, V.,** Carbon disulfide neuropathy in rats. A morphological and ultrastructural study of degeneration and regeneration, *Clin. Toxicol.,* 18, 1463, 1981.

111. **Takahashi, M., Ohara, T., and Hashimoto, K.,** Electrophysiological study of nerve injuries in workers handling acrylamide, *Int. Arch. Arteitsmed.,* 28, 1, 1971.

112. **Gilliatt, R. W., Fowler, T. J., and Rudge, P.,** Peripheral neuropathy in baboons, *Adv. Neurol.,* 10, 253, 1975.

113. **Satchell, P. M., McLeod, J. G., Harper, B., and Goodman, A. H.,** Abnormalities in the vagus nerve in canine acrylamide neuropathy, *J. Neurol. Neurosurg. Psych.,* 45, 609, 1982.

114. **Post, E. J. and McLeod, J. G.,** Acrylamide autonomic neuropathy in the cat. I. Neurophysiological and histological studies, *J. Neurol. Sci.,* 33, 353, 1977.

115. **Sumner, A. J. and Asbury, A. K.,** Acrylamide neuropathy: selective vulnerability of sensory fibers, *Trans. Am. Neurol. Assoc.,* 99, 79, 1974.

116. **Sumner, A. J.,** Preservation of early discharge of muscle afferents in acrylamide neuropathy, *J. Physiol.,* 246, 277, 1975.

117. **Lowndes, H. E., Baker, T., Cho, E.-S., and Jortner, B. S.,** Position sensitivity of de-efferented muscle spindles in experimental acrylamide neuropathy, *J. Pharmacol. Exp. Ther.,* 205, 40, 1978.

118. **Lowndes, H. E. and Baker, T.,** Studies on drug-induced neuropathies. III. Motor nerve deficit in cats with experimental acrylamide neuropathy, *Eur. J. Pharmacol.,* 35, 177, 1976.

119. **Hopkins, A. P. and Lambert, E. H.,** Conduction in unmyelinated fibers in experimental neuropathy, *J. Neurosurg. Psych.,* 35, 163, 1972.

120. **Von Burg, R., Penney, D. P., and Conroy, P. J.,** Acrylamide neurotoxicity in the mouse: a behavioral electrophysiological and morphological study, *J. Appl. Toxicol.,* 1, 227, 1981.

121. **Baker, T. and Lowndes, H. E.,** Muscle spindle function in organo-phosphorus neuropathy, *Brain Res.,* 185, 77, 1980.

122. **Lowndes, H. E., Baker, T., and Riker, W. F.,** Motor nerve dysfunction in delayed DFP neuropathy, *Eur. J. Pharmacol.,* 29, 66, 1974.

123. **Sedal, L., Ghabriel, M. N., Allt, G., LeQuesne, P. M., and Harrison, M. G.,** A combined morphological and electrophysiological study of conduction block in peripheral nerve, *J. Neuro. Sci.,* 60, 293, 1983.

124. **Chen, R. C., Chang, Y. C., Chang, K. J., Lu, F. J., and Tung, T. C.,** Periphenal neuropathy caused by chronic polychlorinated biphenyls poisoning, *J. Formosan Med. Assoc.,* 80, 47, 1981.

125. **Seppalainen, A. M. and Hakkinen, I.,** Electrophysiological findings in diphenyl poisoning, *J. Neurol. Neurosurg. Psych.,* 38, 248, 1975.

126. **Guiheneuc, P., Ginet, J., Groleau, J. Y., and Rojouan, J.,** Early phase of vincristine neuropathy in man with transitory enhancement of spinal transmission of the monosynaptic reflex, *J. Neurol. Sci.,* 45, 355, 1980.

127. **Bosch, E. P., Pelham, R. W., Rosool, C. G., Chatterjee, A., Lash, R. W., Brown, L., Munsat, T. L., and Bradley, W. G.,** Animal models of alcoholic neuropathy: morphologic, electrophysiologic, and biochemical findings, *Muscle Nerve,* 2, 133, 1979.

Chapter 8

SENSORY NERVE TERMINAL FUNCTION

Barry D. Goldstein

TABLE OF CONTENTS

I.   Introduction 72

II.   Nomenclature of Primary Sensory Fibers and Their Innervation 72
       A.   Sensory Afferents 72
       B.   Sensory Receptors 72
             1.   Muscle Receptors 72
                   a.   Muscle Spindles 72
                   b.   Golgi Tendon Organs 74
                   c.   Mechanoreceptors 74
             2.   Cutaneous Receptors 74
                   a.   Mechanoreceptors 74
                   b.   Thermoreceptors 76
                   c.   Nocireceptors 76
             3.   Joint Receptors 76
             4.   Visceral Receptors 76

III.   Toxicology of Peripheral Sensory Terminals 76
       A.   Proprioceptor Function 77
             1.   Chemicals 77
             2.   Drugs 78
             3.   Animal Toxins 79
       B.   Cutaneous Receptor Function 79
             1.   Chemicals 79
             2.   Drugs 80

IV.   Methodology 80
       A.   Muscle Spindle Activity 80
             1.   General Procedures 80
             2.   Stimulating and Recording Techniques 81
             3.   Conduction Velocity Determination 82
             4.   Measurement of Muscle Spindle Position and Velocity
                   Sensitivity 82
       B.   Cutaneous Mechanoreceptors 82

V.   Summary 84

Acknowledgment 84

References 84

I. INTRODUCTION

The peripheral nervous system is a primary site of action for many toxins. This is primarily due to the lack of a protective barrier like the blood-brain barrier. This chapter deals with the effects of toxins on sensory nerve terminal function. While it is not the intent of this chapter to present a review of the physiology of the sensory nerve terminal, some physiology is necessary in order to comprehend the methodologies and pathophysiology.

The primary sensory neuron is a unipolar neuron with the cell body located in the dorsal root ganglia (see Figure 1). It has two processes arising from the cell body. One process extends to the peripheral nervous system and innervates the skin, muscle, and viscera. The other process travels centrally and terminates in the spinal cord. The primary sensory neuron has two sensory nerve terminals, a peripheral nerve ending, which receives information from sensory receptors and, a central terminal which transmits the information received from the sensory receptors. For the purpose of this chapter, I will only be discussing the peripheral sensory nerve terminal. The central sensory nerve terminal will be discussed elsewhere.

II. NOMENCLATURE OF PRIMARY SENSORY FIBERS AND THEIR INNERVATION

A. Sensory Afferents

Most peripheral nerves are composed of both sensory and motor axons. The sensory nerves can be divided into two major types, cutaneous and muscle. Some peripheral nerves are solely cutaneous or muscle while others contain both types of sensory nerves. The nomenclature for cutaneous nerves is alphabetic and for muscle afferents it is numeric. Visceral nerves and nerves innervating the joints are also alphabetic. The largest-diameter fibers in cutaneous nerves are Aα and Aβ.[19] They have conduction velocities ranging from 30 to 100 m/sec. The small mylineated fibers are Aδ fibers and the unmylineated fibers are C fibers. these afferents conduct at 4 to 30 m/sec and less than 2.5 m/sec, respectively. Muscle afferents are divided into groups I, II, and III, which are mylineated,[4,43] and group IV afferents, which are unmylineated.[55] These afferents conduct at 72 to 100 m/sec for group I, 24 to 71 m/sec for group II, 6 to 23 m/sec for group III, and less than 2.5 m/sec for group IV.[31]

B. Sensory Receptors

The peripheral sensory afferent innervates the sensory receptor. These sensory receptors are normally grouped by their location, i.e., skeletal muscle, skin, joints, and viscera.

1. Muscle Receptors

Skeletal muscle has several types of sensory receptors. They include proprioceptors (muscle spindles and golgi tendon organs) and mechanoreceptors (Pacinian corpuscles and those relaying deep pressure and pain). The structure and function of muscle receptors has been reviewed in detail by Matthews.[47] However, for clarity, a brief description of these receptors is necessary.

a. Muscle Spindles

The muscle spindles are proprioceptors which play a critical role in coordinated muscle movements and reflex activity.[47] They consist of several intrafusal fibers contained in a capsule.[26] Stretch of the parent extrafusal muscle also results in parallel length changes in the intrafusal muscle fibers, histologically classified as nuclear bag or nuclear chain fibers according to the appearance of their nuclei.[9] The nuclear bag fibers are innervated by annulospiral endings (primary endings) which give rise to group Ia afferent fibers. The nuclear chain fibers are innervated by both primary endings and flower-spray (secondary)

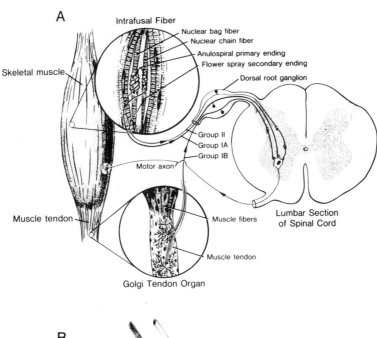

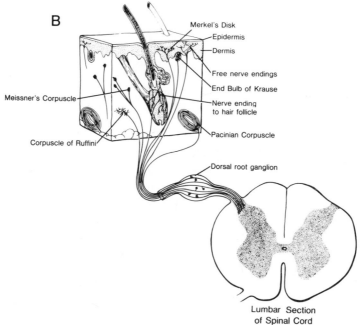

FIGURE 1.   Diagram of proprioceptive (A) and cutaneous (B) sensory terminals, their innervation and termination in the spinal cord. (A) Muscle showing intrafusal fiber (inset) and Golgi tendon organ (inset). See text for explanation. (B) Cross section of skin showing the different types of cutaneous receptors. See text for explanation.

endings which synapse in the spinal cord via group II afferent fibers.[5,9] Figure 1A shows a drawing of the muscle spindle and its innervation. The primary endings are sensitive to both the velocity and length of stretch of muscles. Upon stretch of a muscle (ramp and hold) a brief, high-frequency burst of action potentials (phasic discharge) is generated, followed by a slower, largely maintained discharge (statis discharge). Peak frequency of the phasic burst of action potentials is proportional to the rate of change of muscle length while the frequency ot the static discharge is proportional to the length of the muscle.[47] The velocity sensitivity of the muscle is measured by the dynamic index, defined as the difference between the peak dynamic frequency and the frequency of discharge 0.5 sec after stretch is initiated.[16] The secondary endings respond primarily to muscle length and hence their discharge provides an index of position sensitivity of the muscle spindle ending. Position sensitivity is determined from the slope of the relationship between the length of the muscle and the frequency of discharge of the muscle spindle endings.[18,27,36]

Both nuclear bag and chain fibers are innervated by fusimotor (gamma efferents) fibers.[5,9] Activation of these efferent fibers causes contraction of intrafusal muscle fibers and thus enhances the sensitivity of the muscle to change in the length of the parent extrafusal muscle.

The impulses generated by the primary endings, whose afferent fiber diameters range from 12 to 20 μm, are conducted at 72—120 m/sec.[31] These Ia afferents make monosynaptic connection with α-motoneurons (α-MN) innervating the homonymous muscle (Figure 1A)[47] and other spinal cord synapses. The impulses initiated in secondary endings, whose fiber diameters range from 6 to 12 μm, are conducted at 20 to 72 m/sec by group II axons. These group II fibers make polysynaptic connections with α-MNs innervating the homonymous muscle (Figure 1A).[47]

b. Golgi Tendon Organs

Golgi tendon organs are also proprioceptors. However, unlike muscle spindles, they respond to contraction of the muscle.[30] Tendon organs usually lie at the junction of the muscle and tendon (Figure 1A).[4] They reside at both the origin and insertion. They are innervated by large-diameter myelineated afferents (group Ib). The group Ib afferents make polysynaptic connections in the spinal cord and are responsible for autogenetic inhibition.[47] Stimulation of group Ib afferents inhibit extension muscles and excites flexor muscles. Therefore, it appears that Golgi tendon organs are responsible for the "protection" of the muscle from too much contraction.

c. Mechanoreceptors

Skeletal muscle also contains a number of mechanoreceptors. They respond to vibration (Pacinian corpuscle; infra vida), deep pressure (medulated free nerve endings; group III afferents),[48] and pain (nonmedulated free nerve endings; group IV afferents).[33]

2. Cutaneous Receptors

Receptors in the skin transmit a variety of sensory modalities including mechanoreception (tactile), thermoreception, and nociception. The characteristics of these receptors has been extensively reviewed elsewhere;[11] however, it is necessary to provide a brief description of these receptors for background for the toxicological studies and methods. Table 1 is a summary of the characteristics of the major types of cutaneous sensory receptors.

a. Mechanoreceptors

Mechanoreceptors are most readily activated by some form of mechanical change in the skin. There are several types of mechanoreceptors and they can be characterized by the way they respond to a mechanical stimulus. There are receptor types which respond to displacement and velocity alone, and acceleration.[29]

The receptors which respond to displacement and velocity are called slowly adapting Type I (SA1) and type II (SA2) receptors.[11] SAI receptors are associated with Merkel cell receptors which are also known as touch dome receptors or Haarscheibs (Figure 1B).[34,52] The SA1 has little or no resting discharge and possesses both position and dynamic sensitivities, i.e., it will respond to velocity changes and displacement changes. Figure 2 shows the neuronal response of an SA1 receptor to a displacement of 500 μm and a velocity of 5 μm/msec.

Table 1
CRITERIA FOR IDENTIFICATION FOR CUTANEOUS MECHANORECEPTORS

Mechanoreceptor type	Mean conduction velocity (m/sec)	Type of response	General receptive field
SA1	65	Velocity and prolonged displacement; irregular discharge	Punctate
SA2	65	Velocity and prolonged displacement; regular discharge; responds to stretch	Punctate
Field	50—65	Velocity only	Widespread
Rapidly adapting	60—65	Velocity only	Punctate

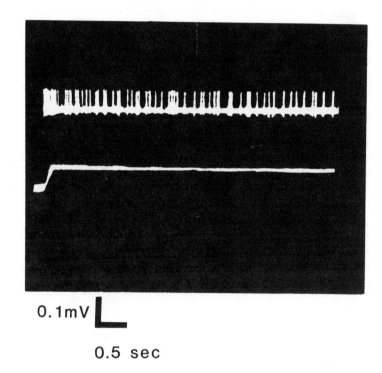

0.1mV

0.5 sec

FIGURE 2.   Oscilloscope tracing of the discharge pattern of a SA1 receptor. Lower trace is the ramp and hold stimulus waveform. Upper trace is the actual recording. Note the initial velocity component during the ramp stimulus and the prolonged irregular pattern during the hold pattern of the stimulus. Ramp is 5 mm/sec and hold is 500 μm displacement.

Note the initial burst of activity followed by a steady irregular discharge. This is characteristic for an SA1 receptor. The discharge will continue for over 100 sec.

SA2 receptors are associated with Ruffini endings (Figure 1B). They respond to velocity and displacement; however, unlike SA1 receptors, SA2 receptors have a resting discharge, can be excited by stretch of the skin, and, during the steady (static) discharge of the receptors, show a very regular pattern.

There are several types of velocity detectors. These include hair follicle receptors, field receptors, and rapidly adapting receptors. Hair follicle receptors respond to the velocity of hair movement (Figure 1B). Continual or maintained stimulation of the hair receptors will not produce a sustained response.[12] Field receptors are velocity sensors but respond to stimulation over wide areas of the skin.[60] The sense organ of the field receptor is unknown.

In glaborous skin there are also velocity receptors known as rapidly adapting receptors (RA). RA receptors are associated with Krause's end-bulbs in cat footpad[35] and Meissner's corpuscles in primate skin (Figure 1B).[49] The RA receptors respond to velocity; however, their receptive field is very distinct or punctuate.

A third category of mechanoreceptors is the transient or accleration detector, the most common of which is the Pacinian corpuscle (Figure 1B). Pacinian corpuscles are transient detectors. They are very sensitive with thresholds of less than 1 μm[32] and respond best to vibration frequencies of 60 to 300 Hz.[59] They are located in skin, muscle, and viscera.

b. Thermoreceptors

There are two kinds of thermoreceptors in the skin which convey innocuous changes of temperature. They are cold and warm receptors. Cold receptors are associated with free nerve endings, have a resting discharge, and respond by increasing their rate of firing to both dynamic and static changes.[17] The dynamic response signals the rate at which the temperature changes and the static response signals the temperature level.

Warm receptors are presumed to be associated with free nerve endings and have a resting discharge. They respond by accelerating their discharge with warming (maximum at 45°C) and decrementing their discharge with cooling.[28]

c. Nociceptors

There are several types of receptors which convey the modality of pain. They are associated with free nerve endings and are innervated by Aδ and C fibers. Aδ nociceptors which respond to mechanical stimulation are excited best by mechanical damage to the skin. They do not respond to noxious heat, cold, or chemical irritation.[10] C fiber mechanical nociceptors respond similarly to the Aδ receptors.[6] Aδ and C thermoreceptors are divided into two types, heat and cold. The heat receptors respond to noxious heat (>45°C) and noxious mechanical stimuli.[22] The cold receptors respond to extreme cold and noxious mechanical stimuli.[21,23] Polymodal nociceptors are innervated by C fibers and respond to noxious thermal, mechanical, and chemical stimuli.[6]

3. Joint Receptors

Joints contain both slowly adapting receptors and rapidly adapting receptors. The slowly adapting receptors are Golgi tendon organs and Ruffini endings.[8] The rapidly adapting receptors are the paciniform mechanoreceptors. The Golgi tendon organs and paciniform receptors respond as described above. The Ruffini endings appear to signal changes in the torque that is developed as the joint is moved.[13,15]

4. Visceral Receptors

The viscera contain mechanoreceptors (Pacinian corpuscles), nociceptors, and thermoreceptors. These receptors all respond in a similar manner as those described previously.

III. TOXICOLOGY OF PERIPHERAL SENSORY TERMINALS

The major neurological sequalae associated with neurotoxic agents are ataxia, loss of reflexes, parathesias, and numbness.[2,14,20,38,40,50,58] These sequalae can be attributed to loss of function in any number of places in the peripheral and central nervous systems. A systematic experimental protocol is usually followed to determine what neural substrates are affected and the temperospatial involvement of these neural substrates.

Usually, sensory terminal function is studied because of the obvious involvement of sensory receptors in the elaboration of the above-mentioned sequalae.

There have been three major types of studies on the effects of toxic substances on sensory receptors. The simplest is the characterization of the afferent discharge and then determining whether the receptor is active or not. These studies are "all or none" studies, i.e., they tell you whether the receptors or afferent fibers have been destroyed by the toxin. They do not tell you whether the ones which are present are functioning normally. The more complex and comprehensive studies are those which not only determine whether the receptor is present but also construct tuning curves or frequency-response relationships. These studies will tell the physiological condition of those receptors which are present. However, these studies cannot distinguish between damage to the receptor generator potential or damage to the preterminal or terminal part of the afferent fiber. The third type of study actually records the generator potential and can determine whether that part of the transduction mechanism is functioning normally.

A. Proprioceptor Function

The majority of the toxicological studies performed on proprioceptive function have been on muscle spindle primary and secondary endings. I have categorized these types of toxicological studies as the effects of (1) chemicals, (2) drugs, and (3) animal toxins on muscle spindle function.

1. Chemicals

The neurotoxic chemicals which have been shown to affect muscle spindle function are acrylamide[44,45,56,57] and organophosphorous compounds.[3]

Acrylamide is a vinyl monomer ($CH_2 = CH\ CONH_2$) which is neurotoxic. It produces a classical central-peripheral distal axonopathy.[53] The rationale for the study of acrylamide on muscle spindle function is that poisoning causes ataxia and loss of deep tendon reflexes in man and experimental animals. Also, morphological data suggest that sensory processes are involved prior to motor processes.[51] Thus, several studies have been undertaken to determine whether proprioceptors are involved and if so, the exact nature of the dysfunction.[44,45,56,57]

Sumner and Asbury[56,57] were the first investigators to determine that there was in fact a defect in muscle spindle and Golgi tendon organ function. They isolated medial gastrocnemius muscle afferents by stimulating the gastrocnemius nerve and recording from L_7 dorsal root fibers in the spinal cord. Following isolation of the afferent, they determined whether the unit was an annulospiral ending, a flower-spray ending, or a Golgi tendon organ. This was determined by conduction velocity and response to contraction and stretch of the muscle. Sumner and Asbury[56,57] divided the animals into three groups. Each animal received 10 mg/kg/day acrylamide. Group A received a total of 210 to 340 mg/kg (21 to 34 days); group B received a total of 380 to 440 mg/kg (38 to 44 days); group C received 470 to 670 mg/kg. The animals showed mild, moderate, and severe clinical signs of the neurotoxicity. The investigators found that in group A 10% of the afferents would not respond to stretch or contraction; 68% were nonresponsive in group B and 89% in group C. The weaknesses of this study were that the investigators did not have a group of control animals to determine how many nonresponsive afferent normally occur with this technique. Similar studies on vincristine (see below) have shown that in normal cat soleus muscle 65% of the afferents are responsive muscle spindles. It was also possible that some of the nonresponsive afferents they recorded were from paciniform corpuscles and were not activated by the stimuli they used. Furthermore, there was no way of knowing whether or not the responding units were functioning in the normal physiological range.

Further and more complete studies on muscle spindle function were then carried out.[44,45] Lowndes and co-workers[44,45] performed a series of experiments to determine whether annulospiral or primary endings and flower-spray or secondary endings were functioning normally following chronic acrylamide exposure. In the first study,[44] they tested the position sensitivity or static response of primary and secondary endings. They set up three treatment groups of 7.5, 15, and 30 mg/kg/day; 10 days was the maximum number of days animals received acrylamide. There were animals in the 15 and 30 mg/kg/day group which were studied prior to the 10 days and those which were allowed 1 to 5 weeks recovery time prior to being studied. The investigators found no change in afferent conduction velocity but did find changes in muscle spindle function. Both primary and secondary endings displayed elevated thresholds, i.e., the amount of muscle stretch necessary to produce a static or continuous discharge. They also found that at any given stretch the discharge frequency was reduced. These changes were found to occur as early as 4 days after 15 mg/kg/day in secondary endings and 7 days after 15 mg/kg/day in primary endings. Recovery from these effects occurred slowly and incompletely.

The second study[45] tested the dynamic response or velocity sensitivity of solely primary endings (since secondary endings have little or no dynamic response) following acrylamide treatment. Cats were exposed to 30 mg/kg/day of acrylamide for 5 or 10 days. Velocity sensitivity of control and the two treated groups was determined by stretch of the soleus muscle at known velocities (10, 20, and 40 m/sec) to a constant position. The dynamic index (peak frequency during velocity component minus static component) was determined. The investigators found that the velocity sensitivity of primary endings was depressed following 10 days but not 5 days of acrylamide treatment. This coincided with the neurological changes of hard to elicit tendon reflexes. Since the velocity sensitivity is in part responsible for tendon reflexes and position sensitivity for coordination, these two studies have shown that muscle spindle dysfunction plays an important part in the elaboration of the neurological sequalae following acrylamide administration.

Organophosphorous agents is another group of compounds which have been studied for changes in muscle spindle function. Certain organophosphorus agents have been shown to produce a delayed neurotoxicity with neurological sequalae consisting of ataxia, loss of reflexes, and muscle weakness.[14] Baker and Lowndes[3] have shown that localized injections of diisopropylfluorophosphate (DFP) produced a mononeuropathy which affects muscle spindle function. The investigators found that the position sensitivity of both primary and secondary endings was affected, but that secondary endings were damaged prior to the primary endings. The similarity to acrylamide is that secondary endings appear more sensitive than primary endings. However, unlike acrylamide, where sensory terminal function is depressed prior to motor terminal, in organophosphorus neuropathy the motor nerve terminal dysfunction occurs at the same time as the sensory nerve terminal dysfunction.

However, not all organophosphorus agents will damage muscle spindle terminals. Goldstein[24] has shown that muscle spindle primary and secondary endings have normal position sensitivities following treatment with soman, a potent acetylcholinesterase (AChE) inhibitor.

2. Drugs

Certain drugs have been shown to affect muscle spindle activity as a side effect of that agent. In particular, ethanol, vincristine, and steroids[7,24,38,39,41] have been shown to alter proprioceptive function.

Ethanol is a depressant drug which impairs motor coordination. Several studes have been performed to determine what effects ethanol has on muscle spindle function.[38,39,41] Smith and co-workers have found that acute administration of ethanol increases the discharge rate of muscle spindle afferents. In vitro application of ethanol caused a biphasic response. At low doses, a concentration-dependent increase in the firing rate of muscle spindles occurred. The lowest effective concentration was 17 mM. This increase in firing rate occurred without the application of stretch. At high concentrations, the firing rate was depressed. They also found that the application of an initial stretch would make the ethanol less effective in increasing the firing rate of the muscle afferent. Systemic administration of ethanol had similar effects.[39] Ethanol (2.5 g/kg i.p.) was administered and the response of triceps surae muscle afferents was recorded. Kucera and Smith found that ethanol, just as in the in vitro application, increased the firing rate of the muscle spindles. They also found that rats exhibited motor impairment at this dose of ethanol.

In studies on cats, Lathers and Smith[41] found similar changes in muscle spindle activities which correlated with the appearance of classical signs of ethanol toxicity.

Steroids also have toxic effects on muscle spindles.[7] Botterman and co-workers[7] found that the administration of triamcinolone (4 mg/kg) for 10 to 12 days produced a greater number of spontaneously firing spindles and a decreased length threshold in nonspontaneously firing units. A decrease in position sensitivity was also found. Since steroids induce skeletal muscle atrophy, the authors suggest that these changes are related to damage to the muscular component of the spindle rather than damage to the sensory nerve terminal itself.

Finally, vincristine, an antineoplastic agent, has been shown to affect muscle spindle activity. Vincristine is a vinca alkaloid which inhibits mitotic spindles and causes neurofilamentous accumulation in nervous tissue. It produces a peripheral neuropathy which is different from that produced by acrylamide and other chemical agents. Goldstein et al.[24] administered 50 μg/kg vincristine i.v. every 4 days until classical signs of the neuropathy appeared (ataxia, loss of reflexes, muscle weakness). Muscle spindle position and velocity sensitivity was assessed along with a count of the number of muscle receptors encountered. They found that approximately 80% of the afferent units were unresponsive to any form of muscle stimulus (contraction or stretch). Investigations into the response characteristics of the responsive spindle showed depressed dynamic sensitivities of primary endings but no change in the position sensitivity of either primary or secondary endings.

3. Animal Toxins

The major reason for discussing the effects of animal toxins, in particular tetrodotoxin (TTX), is because of the technique used to show the toxic effects of TTX on sensory terminal function. The technique used enabled the study of the sensory terminal generator potential which elicits the action potentials in the nerve fiber.[1]

TTX is a toxin found in the puffer fish located around Japan. It has been shown to be a very potent sodium ion channel blocker,[1] and in these studies has been used to determine the ionic mechanism of the receptor potential in the muscle spindle. These investigators found that TTX will block the action potential at concentrations of 0.8 to 1.0×10^{-7} g/mℓ but has no effect on the generator potential. This suggests that the generator potential utilizes a different ionic mechanism than the afferent fiber. This ionic mechanism could be a TTX-resistant Na^+ channel or a separate ion channel altogether.

B. Cutaneous Receptor Function

There are very few studies on the effects on toxic agents on cutaneous sensory receptors. A search of the literature shows a total of four studies.[23,24,42,54]

1. Chemicals

Spencer and co-workers[54] have shown that Pacinian corpuscles are damaged following acrylamide pretreatment. In normal animals, Spencer et al. found that 90% of the Pacinian corpuscles isolated from cat mesentery were responsive to mechanical pulses. However, following acrylamide administration, only 41% of the Pacinian corpuscles isolated showed generator potentials and of this 41%, all the units from cats who received greater than 60 mg/kg acrylamide (total dose) were nonresponsive to mechanical stimuli.

In another study using acrylamide as the toxin, Goldstein[25] found that cutaneous mechanoreceptors were affected. Goldstein isolated four types of cutaneous mechanoreceptors: field (F), rapidly adapting (RA), slowly adapting type 1 (SA1), and slowly adapting type 2

(SA2). Frequency-response curves were generated only for SA1 receptors. It was found that the units which were responsive had normal position sensitivity. However, the total number of all types of responsive units was 60% of control. Furthermore, there appeared to be a receptor distribution change. The acrylamide-treated cats had an increase in RA receptors from 16 to 30% and a decrease in SA1 and SA2 receptors from 17 to 3% and 5 to 0%, respectively. This distribution change is probably the result of the SA1 and SA2 receptors having no position sensitivity, thus appearing to be RA receptors.

Goldstein[24] also performed another study on the effects of soman on mechanoreceptor activity. In this study, it was found that subacute administration of soman had no effect on frequency-response curves but did reduce the number of responsive units 66% of control. These data were similar to the acrylamide data; however, there was no apparent change in the distribution of receptor types. This suggests a nonspecific effect on these mechanoreceptors — unlike acrylamide which appear to affect slowly adapting receptors.

2. Drugs

Vincristine has recently been shown to affect SA1 mechanoreceptors.[42] Leon and McComas have shown that a single dose of 0.75 mg/kg vincristine will elevate the threshold for firing of these receptors from 5.2 μm displacement to 14.2 μm. Concomitantly, the discharge of these receptors became less regular and at a given stimulus responded with a lower frequency. These changes are clearly the result of a toxic effect of vincristine on these SA1 receptors. However, it is unclear as to whether these changes are the result of the neuropathic effects of vincristine.

IV. METHODOLOGY

This section will describe in detail some of the techniques used to determine sensory nerve terminal function. Since there are many different techniques, some much more difficult than others, I have chosen those techniques which have been used frequently in the literature. The microelectrode studies of generator potentials are very similar to the studies reported elsewhere in this book and are not discussed.

A. Muscle Spindle Activity

The techniques I will be describing have been used in studies discussed in the previous section.[24,44,45,56,57]

1. General Procedures

Adult cats weighing from 2 to 4 kg can be anesthetized with either sodium pentobenbital (35 mg/kg), α-chloralose (80 mg/kg, i.v.), or a combination of α-chloralose (60 mg/kg) and urethane (400 mg/kg).

I have found the combination of α-chloralose and urethane to be better than either the pentobarbital or α-chloralose alone. If pentobarbital is used, several additional doses will be necessary and if chloralose alone is used there is difficulty in getting the animal anesthetized and periodically there is a convulsive-like action which is manifested by a jumping of the animal. These problems do not exist with the combination of chloralose and urethane.

A tracheal cannula is inserted and blood pressure can be monitored by a carotid artery cannula. The animal is allowed to breathe on its own. A dorsal laminectomy is performed from vertebrae L-3 to S-2. The dura mater is opened longitudinally and the spinal cord exposed. The L_7 and S_1 dorsal and ventral roots are cut proximal to where they enter the spinal cord. L_7 and S_1 are used since it contains the majority of the hindlimb innervation. The ventral roots are cut so that there is no α-motor nerve influence on the muscle spindles.

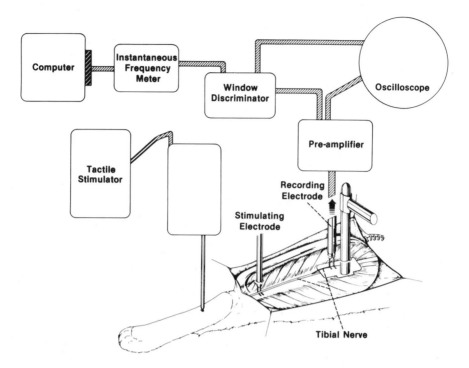

FIGURE 3.   Recording setup for the study of cutaneous sensory receptors. See text for explanation.

Muscle spindles have been isolated from the triceps surae muscle group (medial and lateral gastrocnemius, plantaris, and soleus), the gastrocnemius alone and the soleus alone. There is no real reason why one is used over the other. My preference is the soleus because it is easy to isolate, there are more muscle spindles in it than the gastrocnemius, and it is easier to stretch with a myograph. Therefore, I will discuss the isolation of the soleus muscle and nerve.

The soleus muscle is best isolated in the hindlimb by removal of the biceps, lateral and medial gastrocnemius, and plantaris muscles. The common peroneal and tibial nerve are cut. This leaves the soleus muscle and its innervation intact. Complete deafferentation of the hindlimb is necessary so that the only activity recorded in the dorsal roots is from the soleus afferents. Deafferentation is accomplished by crushing the innervation to the following muscles: caudal femoris, gluteus maximus, gluteus medius, and pyriformis. The calcaneous is cut at the heel so that the soleus muscle can be attached to a myograph.

Surgical pins are inserted in the ankle and knee so that the leg can be kept rigid. The animal is placed in a spinal unit and the skin flaps from both surgical cavities are tied back to make oil pools. The cavities are filled with mineral oil and maintained at 37°C.

2. Stimulating and Recording Techniques

The calcaneous is attached to a force displacement transducer which is connected to a modified Brown-Schuster myograph. Figure 3 shows the recording setup. The intact soleus nerve is placed over a bipolar platinum wire stimulating electrode. The soleus nerve is stimulated with supramaximal square wave pulses of 0.1 msec duration every 2.5 sec (0.4 Hz). A plexiglass platform is placed in the laminectomy with the dorsal root resting on it. This platform aids in the teasing of the dorsal roots to filaments with jeweler's forceps. Responses are recorded from the dorsal root filaments with shielded bipolar platinum wire electrodes. The recording electrode is coupled to a preamplifier (AC recording bandpass 0.3 to 30K Hz). The amplified signals are shunted to an oscilloscope for display.

3. Conduction Velocity Determination

Afferent nerve conduction velocities can be determined by recording the latency of the evoked response from the soleus nerve to the dorsal root filament. At the end of the experiment the nerve is surgically removed and the distance between the stimulating and recording electrodes is measured. The conduction velocity can then be determined by dividing the length (millimeters) by the latency (milliseconds).

4. Measurement of Muscle Spindle Position and Velocity Sensitivity

Position and velocity sensitivity are determined using the techniques described by Harvey and Matthews[27] and Matthews.[46] Both dorsal and ventral roots are cut proximally. Primary and secondary endings are identified in dorsal root filaments by their conduction latencies and their characteristic responses to soleus muscle contraction evoked by indirect stimulation. Primary endings exhibit a silent phase when the muscle is released from stretch (unloading).[47] The secondary endings do not exhibit unloading but decrement their discharge frequency.[47] The discharge characteristics of single afferent fibers is aided by the use of an amplitude discriminator, particularly in filaments containing several active afferents. Once a spindle is isolated and identified, it is tested for either its position or velocity sensitivity.

Position sensitivities of primary and secondary endings are determined by recording their static discharge frequencies during extension of the soleus muscle. The static responses are elicited by stretching the muscle in 2-mm increments every 5 sec to a total of 14 mm. Slack position (0 mm) is determined by stretching the muscle until a deflection of the pen from a polygraph recording (at high gain) shows initial application of tension to the muscle. Static responses are determined by measuring the discharge frequency 0.5 sec after application of each 2-mm stretch increment. The first 0.5 sec of stretch record the velocity component. Discharge frequencies at individual stretch increments are pooled. These responses can be digitized by a computer or a frequency to voltage converter (rate meter) can be used and the output recorded on a chart recorder.

The velocity sensitivities of primary endings is determined by recording the phasic response of the muscle spindle in dorsal root filaments. The phasic response is elicited by stretching the soleus muscle a known amount at varying velocities using a servo-controlled muscle puller.[37] The muscle is maintained at the applied length for 1 sec, giving a ramp-and-hold stretch. The afferent discharge is recorded as described above. The responses are simultaneously fed into an on-line computer which determines the peak frequency (phasic response), the static frequency, and the dynamic index of each muscle spindle primary ending: the dynamic index is calculated as the difference between the phasic response and the static response 0.5 sec after initiation of muscle stretch.[16] The dynamic indices are pooled at each velocity and the relationship of dynamic index and velocity of stretch is determined.

Velocity sensitivity of secondary ending can not be determined since these endings have little, if any, phasic sensitivity.[47]

Concomitant with these studies or if the equipment is not available for measuring position and velocity sensitivity, a count of the number of receptors responding can be made. This is done by isolating functionally single units and characterizing them into primary or secondary muscle spindles or Golgi tendon organs.

B. Cutaneous Mechanoreceptors

There are several ways to isolate and record mechanoreceptors.[10-13,24,25,42] Burgess and Perl[10,12] have used a very difficult technique utilizing microelectrode recordings from peripheral nerve. The technique described below has been utilized in my laboratory with good results.[24,25]

Cats are anesthetized as described above. The tibial nerve is isolated from the sciatic nerve and adjoining tissue. The tibial nerve is cut distal to the hindpaw and the fascicles

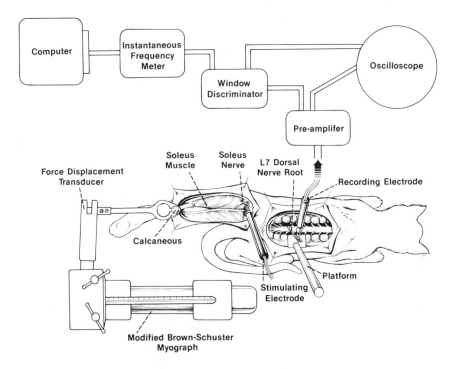

FIGURE 4.   Recording setup for the study of soleus muscle proprioceptors. See text for explanation.

are isolated by removal of the epineurum. The hindpaw is shaved leaving approximately one eigth of an inch to prevent damage to the skin. The skin is further cleaned using a dipilatory. The leg and hindpaw are rigidly mounted with pins at the knee and ankle and the hindpaw braced with wood blocks.

The perineurium is cut and stripped from the fasicle and axons are teased out using jeweler's forceps under microscopic control. Figure 4 shows the setup for recording mechanoreceptors. Small filaments are placed over bipolar platinum hood recording electrode. The recorded signals are amplified and displayed on an oscilloscope. Single units are functionally isolated using an amplitude analyzer and teasing the fibers to very small bundles A stimulating electrode is placed at the distal end of the nerve to record conduction latencies.

Cutaneous tactile receptors are identified by response characteristics, receptive field, and conduction latency.[29] Table 1 shows the identification criteria I have used.

If the identified receptor is an SA1 or SA2 then a frequency-response curve can be generated for displacement. A controlled displacement tactile stimulator is used to accurately activate these receptor types.

The stimulator is of the moving coil or vibrator type and utilizes positional feedback for enhanced response speed and accuracy. It is mounted on an X-Y translation stage for positioning to the area of interest. A z-axis mechanical translator gives coarse control of the stimulus probe height above the skin surface and an electrical position control gives fine adjustment with micron resolution. Probes of different tip shapes and dimensions are easily interchanged by a threaded coupling. The stimulus has a trapezoidal time-displacement waveform with adjustable velocity, duration, and displacement amplitude. The stimulus begins when an external trigger source sets a flip-flop which initiates a positive output from the ramp generator. When the ramp reaches the extension limit set by the plateau amplitude control, it is clamped at that value and triggers a timer whose value is set by the plateau duration control. At the conclusion of the plateau time period, the flip-flop is reset, the ramp generator changes polarity and the probe retracts at the same speed as in the initial segment.

When the probe reaches the baseline position it is again clamped at baseline and the stimulus is complete. The stimulus parameters are adjustable on the front panel and range from 0.1 to 100 mm/sec for extension and retraction speeds, 0 to 1000 μm for plateau amplitude, and 0.1 to 100 sec for plateau duration.

The moving coil actuator drives the probe tip through a coupling that is the magnetic core of a linear variable differential transformer (LVDT). The detected and filtered position signal from the LVDT combines with the output of the ramp generator to produce an error signal that is amplified by the power amplifier to insure that the probe displacement accurately reproduces the desired stimulus waveform. A small (1 μA) current from the continuity detector senses probe tip contact with the skin and a TTL compatible output is provided for triggering an oscilloscope.

For displacement curves, the tactile stimulator is set at a constant velocity (e.g., 5 mm/sec) and plateau duration (at least 10 sec). Displacement is changed anywhere from 5 to 1000 μm.

The unit activity from the amplitude analyzer is directed to an instantaneous frequency meter. The frequency meter determines interspike intervals and converts them to voltages. The output of the frequency meter can be directed to an analogue to digital converted attached on-line to a computer system or it can be directed to a chart recorder and read manually.

The data is processed by plotting the instantaneous frequency against the displacement. The static frequency is defined as the average displacement frequency during the plateau response of the receptor.

A count of the total number of receptors and the receptor type can be performed in a similar way as described above for muscle spindles.

V. SUMMARY

In summary, this chapter has described techniques which can be used to determine functional changes in both proprioceptive and cutaneous sensory receptor terminals. There are other techniques described in the literature in the study of sensory terminal function but they have not yet been used in toxicological studies.[10,12] That is not to say that they are not good for these types of studies, just that the use of these other techniques have not been explored for their contribution to the toxicology data base. I am sure with the expanding field of physiological toxicology these techniques will be utilized.

ACKNOWLEDGMENT

The author wishes to thank Ms. Jennie Doby for her typing of this manuscript. This review as well as some of the cited research was supported by the U.S. Army Medical Research and Development Command DAMD 17-82-C-2217 and NIH grant NS-18664 from NINCDS.

REFERENCES

1. **Albuquerque, E. X., Chung, S. H., and Ottoson, D.,** The action of tetrodotoxin on the frog's isolated muscle spindle, *Acta Physiol. Scand.,* 75, 301, 1969.
2. **Auld, R. B. and Bedwell, S. F.,** Peripheral neuropathy with sympathetic overactivity from industrial contact with acrylamide, *J. Can. Med.,* 96, 652, 1967.
3. **Baker, T. and Lowndes, H. E.,** Muscle spindle function in organophosphorous neuropathy, *Brain Res.,* 185, 77, 1980.

4. **Barker, D.,** The innervation of mammalian skeletal muscle, in *Myotatic Kinesthetic and Vestibular Mechanisms,* deRouck, A. V. S. and Knight, J., Eds., Churchill, London, 1967, 3.

5. **Barker, D. and Hunt, J. P.,** Mammalian intrafusal muscle fibers, *Nature (London),* 203, 1193, 1964.

6. **Bessou, P. and Perl, E. R.,** Response of cutaneous sensory units with ummyelineated fibers to noxious stimuli, *J. Neurophysiol.,* 32, 1025 1969.

7. **Botterman, B. R., Eldred, E., and Edgerton, V. R.,** Spindle discharge in glucocorticoid-induced muscle atrophy, *Exp. Neurol.,* 72, 25, 1981.

8. **Boyd, I. A.,** The histological structure of the receptors in the kneejoint of the cat correlated with their physiological response, *J. Physiol.,* 124, 476, 1954.

9. **Boyd, I. A.,** The structure and innervation of the nuclear bag muscle fibers system and the nuclear chain muscle fibre system in mammalian muscle spindles, *Phil. Trans. R. Soc.,* B245, 81, 1962.

10. **Burgess, P. R. and Perl, E. R.,** Myelinated afferent fibers responding specifically to noxious stimulation of the skin, *J. Physiol.,* 190, 541, 1967.

11. **Burgess, P. R. and Perl, E. R.,** Cutaneous mechanoreceptors and nociceptors, in *Handbook of Sensory Physiology,* Vol. II, Iggo, A., Ed., Springer, New York, 1973.

12. **Burgess, P. R., Petit, D., and Warren, R. M.,** Receptor types in cat hairy skin supplied by myelinated fibers, *J. Neurophysiol.,* 31, 833, 1968.

13. **Burgess, P. R. and Clark, F. J.,** Characteristics of knee joint receptors in the cat, *J. Physiol.,* 203, 317, 1969.

14. **Cavanagh, J. T.,** The significance of the "Dying-back" process in experimental and human neurological disease, *Int. Rev. Exp. Pathol.,* 3, 219, 1964.

15. **Clark, F. J. and Burgess, P. R.,** Slowly adapting receptors in cat knee joint: can they signal joint angle?, *J. Neurophysiol.,* 38, 1448, 1975.

16. **Crowe, A. and Matthews, P. B. C.,** The effects of stimulation of static and dynamic fusimotor fibers on the response to stretching of primary endings of muscle spindles., *J. Physiol.,* 174, 139, 1964.

17. **Darian-Smith, I., Johnson, K. O., and Dykes, R.,** "Cold" fiber population innervating palmar and digital skin of the monkey: response to cooling pulses, *Neurophysiology,* 36, 325, 1973.

18. **Eldred, E., Granit, R., and Merton, P. A.,** Supraspinal control of the muscle spindles and its significance, *J. Physiol.,* 122, 498, 1953.

19. **Erlanger, J. and Gasser, H. S.,** *Electrical Signs of Nervous Activity,* University of Pennsylvania Press, Philadelphia, 1937.

20. **Garland, T. O. and Patterson, M. W. H.,** Six cases of acrylamide poisoning, *J. Br. Med.,* 4, 134, 1967.

21. **Georgopoulos, A. P.,** Functional properties of primary glabrous skin, *J. Neurophysiol.,* 39, 71, 1976.

22. **Georgopoulos, A. P.,** Stimulus-response relations in high-threshold mechanothermal fibers innervating primate glabrous skin, *Brain Res.,* 128, 547, 1977.

23. **Goldstein, B. D., Lowndes, H. E.,and Cho, E.,** Neurotoxicity of vincristine in the cat. Electrophysiological studies, *Arch. Toxicol.,* 48, 253, 1981.

24. **Goldstein, B. D.,** Electrophysiological changes in peripheral sensory receptors following sub-acute administration of soman, *Toxicologist,* 5, 85, 1985.

25. **Goldstein, B. D.,** Acrylamide preferentially affects slowly adapting cutaneous mechanoreceptors, *Toxicol. App. Pharmacol.,* 80, 527, 1985.

26. **Granit, R., Ed.,** *The Basis of Motor Control,* Academic Press, London, 1970.

27. **Harvey, R. J. and Matthews, P. B. C.,** The response of de-efferented muscle spindle endings in the cat's soleus to slow extension of the muscle, *J. Physiol.,* 157, 370, 1961.

28. **Hensel, H. and Kenshalo, D. R.,** Warm receptors in the nasal region of cats, *J. Physiol.,* 204, 99, 1969.

29. **Horch, K. W., Tuckett, R. P., and Burgess, P. R.,** A key to the classification of cutaneous mechanoreceptors, *J. Invest. Dermatol.,* 69, 75, 1977.

30. **Houk, J. and Henneman, E.,** Responses of Golgi tendon organs to active contractions of the soleus muscle of the cat, *J. Neurophysiol.,* 30, 466, 1967.

31. **Hunt, C. C.,** Relation of function to diameter in afferent fibers of muscle nerves, *J. Gen. Physiol.,* 38, 117, 1954.

32. **Hunt, C. C. and McIntrye, A. K.,** Properties of cutaneous touch receptors in cat, *J. Physiol.,* 153, 88, 1960.

33. **Iggo, A.,** Cutaneous mechanoreceptors with afferent C fibers, *J. Physiol.,* 152, 337, 1960.

34. **Iggo, A. and Muir, A. R.,** The structure and function of a slowly adapting touch corpuscle in hairy skin, *J. Physiol.,* 200, 763, 1969.

35. **Iggo, A. and Ogawa, H.,** Correlative physiological and morphological studies of rapidly adapting mechanoreceptors in cats glabrous skin, *J. Physiol.,* 266, 275, 1977.

36. **Jansen, J. K. S. and Matthews, P. B. C.,** The effects of fusimotor activity on the static responsiveness of primary and secondary ending of muscle spindles in the decerebrate cat, *Acta. Physiol. Scand.,* 55, 376, 1962.

37. **Johnson, F. and Murphy, J. T.,** Muscle-pulling system for studies of neural function, *Med. Biol. Eng.,* 11, 78, 1973.
38. **Kucera, J. and Smith, C. M.,** Excitation by ethanol of rat muscle spindles, *J. Pharmacol. Exp. Ther.,* 179, 301, 1971.
39. **Kucera, J. and Smith, C. M.,** Muscle afferent outflow during ethanol intoxication, *Experientia,* 28, 908, 1972.
40. **Kuperman, A. S.,** Effects of acrylmide on the central nervous system of the cat, *J. Pharmacol. Exp. Ther.,* 123, 180, 1958.
41. **Lathers, C. M. and Smith, C. M.,** Ethanol effects on muscle spindle afferent activity and spinal reflexes, *J. Pharmacol. Exp. Ther.,* 197, 126, 1976.
42. **Leon, J. and McComas, A. J.,** Effects of vincristine sulfate on touch dome function in the rat, *Exp. Neurol.,* 84, 283, 1984.
43. **Lloyd, D. P. C. and Chang, H. T.,** Afferent fibers in muscle nerves, *J. Neurophysiol.,* 11, 199, 1948.
44. **Lowndes, H. E., Baker, T., Cho, E., and Jortner, B. S.,** Position sensitivity of de-efferented muscle spindles in experimental acrylamide neuropathy, *J. Pharmacol. Exp. Ther.,* 205, 40, 1978.
45. **Lowndes, H. E., Baker, T., Michelson, L. P., and Vincent-Ablazey, M.,** Attenuated dynamic responses of primary endings of muscle spindles: a basis for depressed tendon responses in acrylamide neuropathy, *Ann. Neurol.,* 3, 433, 1978.
46. **Matthews, P. B. C.,** The response of de-efferented muscle spindle receptors to stretching at different velocities, *J. Physiol.* 168, 660, 1963.
47. **Matthews, P. B. C.,** *Mammalian Muscle Receptors And Their Central Actions,* Williams & Wilkins, Baltimore, 1972.
48. **Paintal, A. S.,** Functional analysis of group III afferent fibers of mammalian muscles, *J. Physiol.,* 152, 250, 1960.
49. **Quilliam, T. A.,** Neuro-cutaneous relationships in fingerprint skin, in *The Somatosensory System,* Kornhuber, H. H., Ed., Thieme, Stuttgart, 1975.
50. **Sandler, S. G., Tobin, W., and Henderson, E. S.,** Vincristine-induced neuropathy, *Neurology,* 19, 367, 1969.
51. **Schaumburg, H. H., Wisniewski, H. M., and Spencer, P. S.,** Ultrastructural studies of the dying-back process. I. Peripheral nerve terminal and axon degeneration in systemic acrylamide intoxication, *J. Neuropathol. Exp. Neurol.,* 33, 260, 1974.
52. **Smith, K. R.,** The Haarscheibe, *J. Invest. Dermatol.,* 69, 68, 1977.
53. **Spencer, P. S. and Schaumburg, H. H.,** Ultrastructural studies of the dying-back process. IV. Differential vulnerability of PNS and CNS fibers in experimental central-peripheral distal axonopathies, *J. Neuropath. Exp. Neurol.,* 36, 300, 1977.
54. **Spencer, P. S., Hanna, R., Sussman, M., and Pappas, G.,** Inactivation of pacinian corpuscle mechanosensitivity by acrylamide, *J. Gen. Physiol.,* 70, 17a, 1977.
55. **Stacey, M. J.,** Free nerve endings in skeletal muscle of the cat, *J. Anat.,* 105, 231, 1969.
56. **Sumner, A. J. and Asbury, A. K.,** Acrylamide neuropathy: selective vulnerability of sensory fibers, *Trans. Am. Neurol. Assoc.,* 99, 79, 1974.
57. **Sumner, A. J. and Asbury, A. K.,** Physiological studies of the dying-back phenomenon, *Brain,* 98, 91, 1975.
58. **Takahashi, M., Ohara, T., and Hashimoto, K.,** Electrophysiological study of nerve injuries in workers handling acrylamide, *Int. Arch. Arbeitmed.,* 28, 7, 1971.
59. **Talbot, W. H., Darian-Smith, I., Kornhaber, H. H., and Mountcastle, V. B.,** The sense of flutter-vibration: comparison of the human capacity with response patterns of mechanoreceptive afferents from the monkey hand, *J. Neurophysiol.,* 31, 301, 1968.
60. **Tuckett, R. P., Horch, K. W., and Burgess, P. R.,** Response of cutaneous hair and field mechanoreceptors in cat to threshold stimuli, *J. Neurophysiol,* 41, 138, 1978.

Chapter 9

MOTOR NERVE ENDING RESPONSIVENESS

Thomas Baker and Herbert E. Lowndes

I.   Introduction 88
      A.   Post-Drug Repetition 88
      B.   Post-Tetanic Repetition 88
      C.   Muscle Response to Post-Drug and Post-Tetanic Repetition 89

II.   Methodology 89
      A.   Anesthesia 90
      B.   Surgical Preparation 90
      C.   Recording Procedures 92

III. Tests of Nerve Terminal Responsiveness in Neurotoxicology 93
      A.   Organophosphate Neuropathy 93
      B.   Systemic Organophosphate Neuropathy 95
      C.   Acrylamide Neurotoxicity 95
      D.   Vincristine 96
      E.   Iminodipropionitrile 96

References 96

Acknowledgments 96

I. INTRODUCTION

The direct recording of electrical events at motor nerve endings is not yet possible due to the minute size of the endings and the limitations of present-day recording techniques. Methods have been developed, however, for indirectly monitoring events which occur at motor nerve endings: one technique is based upon the ability to record potentials and currents from the motor end-plate which reflect prejunctional events and will not be further discussed here (see Chapter 3). A second technique relies on bidirectional impulse conduction following stimulation of peripheral nerves, the orthodromic action potential results in neuromuscular transmission while the antidromic action potential can be recorded from the entire ventral root, from small ventral root filaments which contain only a few axons, or from a single ventral root axon.

A. Post-Drug Repetition

Certain drugs have the capacity to condition motor nerve endings such that a single-action potential invading the endings triggers a train of multiple-action potentials (Figure 1, upper tracings of A,B,C). In this context, the motor nerve ending is that portion of a single myelinated intramuscular axon including the last node of Ranvier and the unmyelinated nerve terminal arborization. The membrane characteristics of the unmyelinated nerve terminal are more like those of a C fiber than those of its larger-diameter, myelinated A fiber intramuscular axon.[1-3] In the presence of drugs like neostigmine or endrophonium, the negative afterpotential of the action potential entering the terminal is greatly enhanced, while that of the intramuscular axon is relatively unaffected. The consequence of this drug action on the motor nerve terminal is that a potential difference is established on the axon; the terminal acts as a negative sink and current flows from the last node of Ranvier to the terminal. If the current is of sufficient strength and duration, the adjoining node is depolarized and a second action potential is generated. It will be conducted antidromically in the intramuscular axon where it can (1) activate (orthodromically) other arborizations innervating other fibers of the motor unit and (2) travel up the axon towards the ventral root. Several antidromic action potentials can be generated at the motor nerve ending by this mechanism, forming a brief repetitive train.

Riker[4] termed agents which cause this sequence of events in motor nerve endings "facilitatory drugs". Facilitatory drugs can cause multiple repetitive firing of endings of motor nerves that innervate either fast or slow mammalian muscle. The recording of facilitatory drug-induced antidromic action potentials in the ventral roots was first described in the early 1940s;[5,6] the technique was independently rediscovered by Riker and co-workers.[7]

B. Post-Tetanic Repetition

A further refinement was developed by Standaert.[8] Cat soleus motor nerve endings are unique in that for a short period of time after conditioning with high-frequency tetanic stimulation, single-action potentials invading the nerve endings are converted to trains of repetitive-action potentials. Again the phenomenon reflects the C fiber-like characteristics of the motor nerve terminal relative to the adjacent myelinated A fiber. After high-frequency conditioning, both the terminal and the nodal regions are hyperpolarized,[8,9] the difference in absolute values of the hyperpolarization establish a sink-source condition between the two regions of the nerve. Subsequent single-action potentials can initiate repetitive firing (Figure 2, upper tracings of A,B,C), analogous to that following conditioning with facilitatory drugs. A limitation of this procedure is that it can be demonstrated only in the cat soleus motor nerve endings. Cat soleus muscle is composed of a homogeneous slow-contracting fiber type which is physiologically distinct from the slow fibers found in mixed muscle.[10]

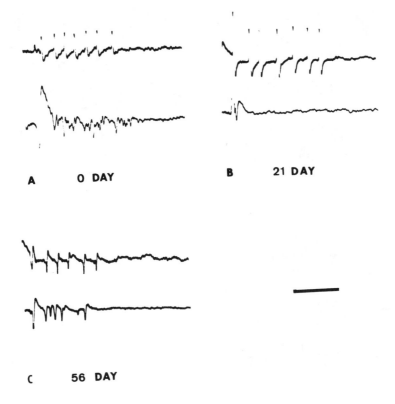

FIGURE 1.   Repetitive discharges generated at cat soleus motor nerve endings conditioned by edrophonium (200 μg/kg i.v.) in a bilateral soleus nerve-muscle preparation: (A) in an untreated control; (B and C) 21 and 56 days, respectively, after unilateral DFP administration. The lower tracings of B and C are recordings made from ventral root axons innervating the soleus muscle of the unilaterally DFP-treated leg. The upper tracing of B and C are recordings from ventral root axons innervating the soleus muscle of the contralateral leg. Time calibration: 10 msec. (From Lowndes, H. E., Baker, T., and Riker, W. F., Jr., *Eur. J. Pharmacol.*, 30, 69, 1975. With permission.)

C. Muscle Response to Post-Drug and Post-Tetanic Repetition

In this in vivo preparation, each stimulus-evoked orthodromic action potential of the nerve initiates the process of neuromuscular transmission, eliciting a contractile response in the innervated muscle. Single supramaximal stimulation of the nerve trunk evokes an almost simultaneous contractile response from all the muscle fibers (the twitch response). The contractile response can be further augmented if the rate of neural stimulation is increased to tetanic frequencies and summation of the muscle responses occur. At the optimal frequency of stimulation, a tetanic tension is developed which can be several times greater than the single maximal muscle response. In this regard, tetanic muscle responses result from either tetanic stimulation or, equally well, from a train of repetitive action potentials triggered in the nerve ending by drug (Figure 3) or tetanic (Figure 4) conditioning.

II. METHODOLOGY

This model was developed using the cat, although in recent studies employing facilitatory drug conditioning, rats have also been used.[11-13] Since this model is not well known, a detailed description of the preparation follows.

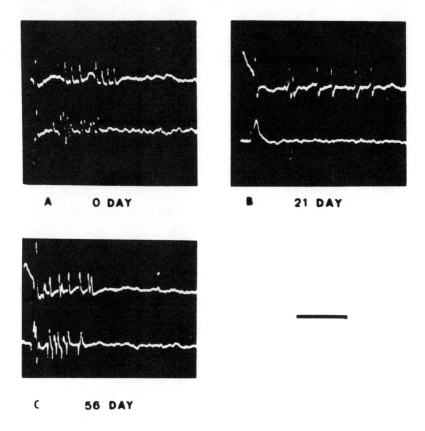

FIGURE 2.   Repetitive discharges generated at cat soleus motor nerve endings generated at cat soleus motor nerve endings conditioned by high frequency stimulation (400 Hz/10 sec) in a bilateral soleus nerve-muscle preparation: (A) in an untreated control; the upper tracings of B and C are recordings made from ventral root axons innervating the soleus muscle of the contralateral leg. The lower tracings of B and C are recordings from ventral root axons innervating the unilateral DFP treated soleus muscle. Time calibration: 20 msec. (From Lowndes, H. E., Baker, T., and Riker, W. F., Jr., *Eur. J. Pharmacol.*, 29, 66, 1974. With permission.)

A. Anesthesia

The anesthesia of choice in cats is α-chloralose, which can be administered either intravenously or intraperitoneally (75 to 90 mg/kg). Chloralose is poorly water soluble, and some researchers made a stock solution by dissolving it in a 20% solution of propylene gycol. This and other organic solvents, however, can affect motor nerve endings function and should not be used. It is preferable to weigh out fresh α-chloralose which is then dissolved in nearly boiling saline and injected after cooling to body temperature. For rats, ethyl carbamate (urethane) provides an excellent surgical anesthesia of sufficient duration. Rats are given two injections of a stock solution (40 gm/100 mℓ of saline): the first, 2 mℓ/kg intraperitoneally, and the second, 1 mℓ/kg subcutaneously, 5 to 10 min later.

B. Surgical Preparation

Following tracheostomy, the hindleg is prepared. A dorsal midline incision is made from the distal end of the ischium to the ankle. The fat pad over the popliteal fossa is removed. The entire fossa is opened and the surface of the gastrocnemius muscle is exposed by blunt dissection. All the nerve rami of the sciatic nerve are ligated and cut, freeing the nerve. The comon peronneal nerve is tied and sectioned just after its origin.

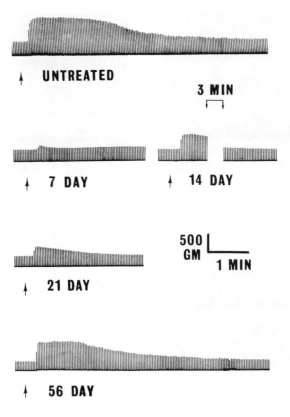

FIGURE 3. The obligatory potentiation of the soleus muscle responses to the repetitive discharges of motor nerve endings conditioned by edrophonium (200 μg/kg i.v. given at arrow). The responses were recorded from muscles of unilaterally DFP treated legs during the course (7 to 56 days) of the neuropathy.

The two heads of the gastrocnemius muscle are gently separated and the trifurcation of the tibial nerve, the only remaining functional nerve bundle in the fossa, is exposed: one branch goes to the lateral head of the gastrocnemius muscle; another goes to the medial head of the gastrocnemius muscle; the last and largest branch, which is the remaining portion of the tibial nerve, extends under the belly of the gastrocnemius muscle. The three branches are gently separated for a short distance (2 to 3 cm), and those not required for the experiment are sectioned.

If a gastrocnemius nerve-muscle preparation is being made, the leg surgery is finished except for making the tendon ready to be connected to a strain gauge. A short incision (approximately 2 to 3 cm) is made over the oscalcis, the heel bone to which the Achilles tendon is connected. The bone is cut with a rib cutter, retaining a small section of the os calcis attached to the Achilles tendon. This facilitates attachment to a keyway slot in a small steel rod, which is connected to a strain gauge.

If a soleus-nerve muscle preparation is being made, further leg surgery is necessary. The gastrocnemius muscle is excised, taking care not to damage the soleus nerve which runs through the lateral head of the gastrocnemius muscle. The gastrocnemius muscle is then excised and the Achilles tendon is prepared for its attachment to the strain gauge rod (see above).

There are three sacral and seven lumbar vertebrae in the cat, and four sacral and six lumbar vertebrae in the rat. An incision is made from vertebra L1 to vertebra S1. The thick,

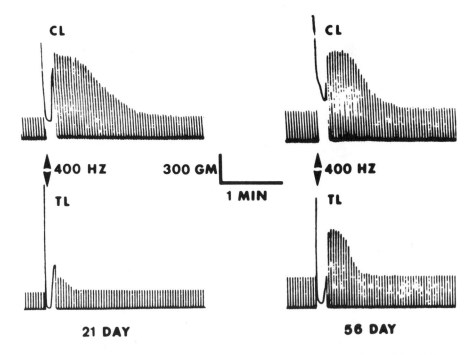

FIGURE 4.   The obligatory potentiation of the soleus muscle responses to the repetitive discharges of motor nerve endings conditioned by high frequency stimulation (400 Hz delivered at arrow for 10 sec) in bilateral soleus nerve muscle preparations at 21 and 56 days after DFP administration. TL: DFP-treated leg. CL: contralateral leg. (From Lowndes, H. E. and Baker, T., *Eur. J. Pharmacol.*, 35, 177, 1976. With permission.)

white sacral fascia which covers the intrinsic spinal column muscles is cut on both sides of the spinal column and the psoas major and minor muscles excised. Intrinsic vertebral muscles are separated from the vertical processes down to and including the dorsal aspects of the horizontal processes from L3 to S3 and then excised. Rongeuring is started at the articulation of L3 and L4 vertebrae. When the spinal cord has been exposed at the articulation, the vertical process of L4 is rongeured and removed. This rongeuring procedure is repeated until all the dorsal portions of the vertebrae down to S1 are removed. At this point the dura is opened, and the ventral roots identified and cut. This procedure can also be done later when the animal is placed in the myograph and the surgical wounds covered with paraffin oil.

C. Recording Procedures

Mounting the animal in a myograph — To record isometric contractile responses of the muscle, the animal is placed in a myograph which holds the leg in a rigid, horizontal position. A modified Brown-Schuster myograph in which the long, heavy bar is placed in a horizontal position is used for cats. There are no commercially available rat myographs. For a gastrocnemius nerve-muscle preparation, a bone pin is passed through the distal head of the femur bone, and for the soleus nerve-muscle preparation, it is passed through the head of the fibula. A second bone pin is passed through the ankle. The pins permit rigid attachment of the leg to the myograph. The skin around the incision forms a pool which is filled with paraffin oil maintained at 37°C. The vertical process of vertebra L3 is attached to a metal frame by means of a spinal clamp. The skin around the laminectomy is used to form another pool which is filled also with heated paraffin oil and is kept at 37°C by radiant heat.

Recording muscle contractile responses — The peripheral soleus nerve is placed on a stimulating electrode which is positioned as close as possible to the entrance of the nerve into the soleus muscle. The nerve is stimulated with supramaximal rectangular pulses of 0.1 msec duration at 0.4 Hz. The strain gauge is adjusted to obtain the isometric twitch in response to supramaximal stimulation.

Recording from the ventral roots — The spinal roots are cut at their exit from the cord if this was not done previously. Each ventral root is placed on a stimulating electrode to determine if a response is evoked in the muscle used in the experiment. The roots are always handled with fine glass hooks. The stimulating parameters can match those used to stimulate the peripheral nerve. Usually both soleus and gastrocnemius nerves are represented in ventral roots S1 and L7 in the cat and L6 and L5 of the rat. Using a fine jeweler's forceps (no. 4 or 5), a root is teased apart into three or four large filaments. Each filament, in turn, is placed on the stimulating electrode to determine its nerve representation by the muscle response. Those filaments having fair to excellent representation are further subdivided. This procedure is repeated until several filaments containing one to four functional axons have been teased out of the larger filaments.

III. TESTS OF NERVE TERMINALS RESPONSIVENESS IN NEUROTOXICOLOGY

The use of techniques for assessing motor nerve terminal responsiveness affords the advantages of establishing the time course and severity of nerve ending involvement in experimental neuropathies; these are valuable correlates of clinical and sensory nerve findings. The original rationale for using these techniques[14] was based on Cavanagh's[15] concept of the "dying-back" process. It was reasoned that if the distal ends of long, large-diameter axons are initially involved in the pathogenesis of toxic neuropathies, functional tests relying on intact motor nerve endings may reveal prodromes or correlates of ensuing axonal degeneration. By extension, quantitation of the tests should provide a measure of extent of motor nerve involvement.[16]

Although the dying-back hypothesis has been modified by subsequent findings,[17] tests of nerve terminal responsiveness have proved useful in establishing the relative and temporal correlations between sensory and motor nerve involvement in organophosphate, acrylamide, and vincristine neurotoxicities. More recent studies with β,β'-iminodipropionitrile (IDPN) further point to the usefulness of the technique; nerve terminal responses are compromised in this model in which axonal atrophy, rather than degeneration, is an eventual outcome.

It should be noted that while these techniques allow sensitive monitoring of nerve terminal function, they remain indirect. As such, they are not capable of addressing questions of mechanisms of neurotoxicity.

A. Organophosphate Neuropathy

Diisopropylfluorophosphate (DFP) mononeuropathy — Lowndes and co-workers[14] developed an exceptional model for a unilateral delayed organophosphorus neuropathy which is produced by the injection of DFP (2 mg/kg) into the femoral artery of a cat's hind leg. This model allows the study of DFP effects on axon and motor nerve endings without compromising the soma or causing the acute cholinergic crisis that occurs with the systemic administration of DFP. The major clinical manifestation of this neuropathy is a peculiar high-step gait of the DFP treated leg caused by tip-toe walking.

Use of the motor nerve ending recording technique[14] in these DFP-treated animals demonstrated that the capacity of soleus motor nerve endings to generate repetitive firing after high-frequency conditioning becomes attenuated 7 days after exposure; the nadir of this motor nerve ending functional loss occurs 21 to 28 days after exposure; after this time, a slow recovery takes place, reaching near complete recovery by 56 days after DFP (Figure 2). At 21 to 23 days after DFP, the percentage of tested axons in the ventral roots from which repetitive firing is recorded is reduced to 9 to 10% from control values of 80 to 83%.[18-20] Nerve conduction velocities are unchanged at the time of the greatest loss of repetitive function of the motor nerve endings.[14]

The obligatory muscle potentiation due to the repetitive discharges of the motor nerve endings after high frequency conditioning is also attenuated in the DFP-treated cats, providing a measure of the functional loss of the repetitive firing capacity of the whole motor nerve ending population.[14] At 21 days after DFP exposure, the obligatory potentiation of the soleus muscle response following high-frequency conditioning of the motor nerve endings is reduced in the unilateral DFP-treated leg to approximately 49% from untreated control values of 194 to 206%.[18,19] The time-course of the muscle potentiation loss and its recovery in the DFP-treated cats correlates with the loss and recovery of the motor nerve ending repetitive function (Figure 4).

Not surprisingly, the ability of facilitatory drugs to generate repetitive firing of the soleus motor nerve endings is also suppressed in DFP neuropathy.[21] A 200 µg/kg intravenous dose of endrophonium, which causes repetitive firing in control animals, fails to have this effect in the DFP neuropathic cats (Figure 1), and the obligatory muscle potentiation due to the facilitatory drug conditioning is also greatly reduced (Figure 3). The time course of the attenuated facilitatory drug effect on motor nerve ending repetitive function and its obligatory muscle potentiation is similar to that of the attenuated responses following high-frequency conditioning. Using this unilateral model, Howland and co-workers[22] found that radiolabeled DFP was distributed in a distal to proximal gradient along the sciatic nerve with the higher radioactivity measurements occurring at the more distal portions of the nerve. The results of this work suggest a direct action of DFP on peripheral nerve and support the findings of the functional studies.

Morphological studies of motor nerve endings from the treated leg of unilateral neuropathic cats show extensive damage occurs at the time of the greatest loss of the repetitive firing capacity of the motor nerve endings.[23,24] DFP induces separate subacute and delayed functional and morphologic changes in the soleus motor nerve endings in this unilateral neuropathy model.[23,25] The subacute damage appears 1 to 3 days after DFP exposure and is confined to the junctional region. While damage is seen in the nerve endings, postjunctional structures are severely involved, and neuromuscular transmission is adversely affected. Both pre- and postjunctional morphological changes are resolved 2 weeks after DFP exposure.

At 3 weeks after DFP exposure, however, the soleus motor nerve endings undergo a delayed degeneration that does not appear related to the earlier pathological events. The most characteristic changes are the presence of large lamellar whorls which often fill entire nerve terminals and are also seen in the intramuscular axons. The membranous material is surrounded by axoplasm. Nerve terminals can be disrupted and retracted from the primary clefts, and the secondary junctional folds are widened.[23,24] Glazer and co-workers[23] examined the neuromuscular junctions of recovering cats exposed to DFP 6 to 8 weeks earlier and found that the majority are nearly or have completely recovered. Thus, a good correlation exists between reestablishment of normal morphology of the nerve endings and the return of repetitive firing in those endings.

Unilateral delayed neuropathy can be prevented by the prior administration of phenyl-methanesulfonyl fluoride.[18] Pretreatment with phenylmethanesulfonyl fluoride (30 mg/kg i.p.) 24 hr before the intraarterial injection of DFP protects cats from the organophosphorus neuropathy. At 21 days after DFP exposure, the time at which unprotected cats demonstrate neurological impairment, no clinical symptoms are observed. The repetitive firing capacity of the soleus motor nerve endings is not lost at this time and its incidence of occurrence approaches normal values. In contrast, only 9% of nerve fibers tested demonstrate repetitive firings in nonprotected DFP animals; in phenylmethanesulfonyl fluoride-protected animals 60% of the axons respond positively, a response much closer to the 83% response found in untreated control cats. The obligatory muscle potentiation following high-frequency conditioning in the phenylmethanesulfonyl fluoride-protected animals also is much greater than that in unprotected cats (168 vs. 47%) and also approaches normal values (206%).

Another study of the phenylmethanesulfonyl protection against the DFP-induced unilateral neuropathy confirmed the preservation of the repetitive firing capacity of motor nerve endings and demonstrated that no morphological changes occur in the nerve endings.[20] Prior treatment with phenylmethanesulfonyl fluoride dramatically prevents any DFP-induced changes in the neuromuscular junctions and intramuscular axons. Although a small fraction of the sampled nerve endings do contain small lamellar whorls, no larger whorls are observed, and 68% of nerve terminals are found to be normal, showing again a good correlation between the degree of structural damage and motor nerve ending repetitive functional loss.

The development of the unilateral delayed neuropathy is prevented by high dose regimens of glucocorticoids given after DFP exposure. An intravenous injection (90 mg/kg) of methylprednisolone given 5 to 10 min after DFP administration followed by 7 intramuscular injections of triamcinolone once every 3 days completely prevents any clinical manifestations of the neuropathy up to 70 days after DFP exposure.[19] Both the incidence of ventral root axons demonstrating repetitive firing originating from motor nerve endings and the obligatory potentiation of the muscle responses are well within the normal control values (78 and 185%, respectively). A similar glucocorticoid regimen employing only methylprednisolone, but one in which the initial intravenous injection was given 30 min after DFP exposure also completely prevents the development of the DFP neuropathy.[26] The percentage of ventral root axons from which repetitive firing is recorded is well within normal control values.

A morphological study of the glucocorticoid-treated DFP animals demonstrated that the steroid regimen prevents any morphological damage.[24] In these animals, over 90% of motor nerve terminals were found to be without evidence of morphological change at 21 to 23 days after DFP administration, the time at which morphological damage is most evident in DFP only treated cats.

B. Systemic Organophosphate Neuropathy

Tri-*ortho*-cresyl phosphate — Although the unilateral model of the organophosphorus neuropathy establishes that motor nerve endings are a site of the neurotoxic effects of DFP, they certainly are not the only possible locus of neurotoxic actions of systemically administered organophosphates. When various neurotoxic agents are administered systemically, they exert their effects on dendrites, soma, axon, and nerve endings. The degree to which each of these sites is affected is determined by the specific agent and the relative vulnerabilities of these neural structures.[27]

Cats which receive subcutaneous tri-*ortho*-cresyl phosphate (1.0 mℓ/kg, 99% purity) develop clinical signs of a systemic neuropathy by 14 days after administration: ataxia and weakness in the hind quarters. By 21 to 28 days following the injection, cats are grossly ataxic and weak, and will not jump even when prodded. Evaluation of the capacity of the soleus motor nerve ending repetitive firing at this time demonstrates great attenuation (6%), similar to that found in the unilateral diisopropylfluorophosphate neuropathic cats. There is no significant change in the motor axonal conduction velocities. The obligatory muscle potentiation following 400 Hz/10 sec conditioning is also greatly reduced.

C. Acrylamide Neurotoxicity

The repetitive firing capacity of soleus motor nerve endings has been assessed in cats which received intramuscular acrylamide (15 mg/kg) daily for 10 days.[16] Tests of the repetitive function of soleus motor nerve endings were carried out 10, 17, 31, and 45 days after the start of acrylamide administration. The percentage of ventral root axons from which repetitive discharges are recorded falls from a control value of 85 to 79%, 71%, 31% and 22% on each respective test day. The obligatory muscle potentiation is also attenuated, reaching the lowest degree of potentiation on test day 45. Motor nerve conduction velocities remain unaffected throughout the study. While this work indicates that an initial functional deficit of motor nerve occurs in the nerve endings, the time-course of this deficit lags well behind the development of the clinical symptoms of this neuropathy which become evident by day 7 of the dosing regimen. At this time, the cats are ataxic, display truncal sway when walking, and are uncoordinated when jumping and landing. In other studies, Lowndes and co-workers[28,29] have demonstrated that the attenuation of motor spindle function does occur in acrylamide-treated cats, and that this attenuation begins contemporaneously with the onset of the clinical symptoms of this neuropathy. Thus, the clinical manifestations and the results of these studies indicate that the sensory nerves are affected earlier than motor axons.

D. Vincristine

Toxic agents may alter sensory nerve function without effect on the repetitive function of motor nerve endings. In cats made neurotoxic by chronic exposure to vincristine (total dose, 300 to 1350 μg/kg), there is no loss of the repetitive discharge capacity of the soleus motor nerve endings or the obligatory potentiation of the soleus muscle responses, although motor nerve conduction velocities are slowed in the neuropathic animals.[30] Clinically, these cats are ataxic and fail to land evenly on their four paws. Achilles tendon reflexes are absent. Muscle spindle function, however, is greatly attenuated in these cats: most primary endings are nonresponsive and the thresholds of position sensitivity of secondary endings are elevated. Sensory nerve conduction velocities are slowed. Morphological studies have shown large swellings in proximal portions of peripheral nerves with only a few swellings occurring in the distal nerve portions. Scattered fibers exhibit Wallerian degeneration, particularly involving larger axons.[31]

E. Iminodipropionitrile

The repetitive firing function of motor nerve endings was also assessed in cats treated with β,β'-iminodipropionitrile (IDPN).[32] IDPN was administered intraperitoneally (50 mg/kg) five times over a 4-week period and the repetitive firing function was assessed 1 week after the last injection. At this time, the cats have become ataxic and walk with their hind legs dragging and set wide apart. In those animals, only 29% of the ventral roots axons display repetitive firing compared to control values of 83%.

ACKNOWLEDGMENTS

The authors' works cited in this article have been supported by USPHS NIH grants NS 01447, NS 11948, NS 23325 and the Amyotrophic Lateral Sclerosis Society of America. The authors also thank Ms. Gail Bahney for her assistance in preparing this manuscript.

REFERENCES

1. **Riker, W. F., Jr. and Standaert, F. G.,** The action of facilitatory drugs and acetylcholine on neuromuscular transmission, *Ann. N.Y. Acad. Sci.,* 135, 163, 1966.
2. **Standaert, F. G. and Riker, W. F., Jr.,** The consequences of cholinergic drug actions on motor nerve terminals, *Ann. N.Y. Acad. Sci.,* 144, 517, 1967.
3. **Riker, W. F., Jr. and Okamoto, M.,** Pharmacology of motor nerve terminals, *Ann. Rev. Pharmacol.,* 9, 173, 1969.
4. **Riker, W. F., Jr.,** Prejunctional effects of neuromuscular blocking and facilitatory drugs, in *Muscle Relaxants,* Katz, R. L., Ed., North-Holland, New York, 1975, 59.
5. **Masland, R. L. and Wigton, R. S.,** Nerve activity accompanying fasciculations produced by prostigmin, *J. Neurolphysiol.,* 3, 269, 1940.

6. **Feng, T. P. and Li, T. H.,** Studies on the neuromuscular junction. XXIV. The repetitive discharges of mammalian motor nerve endings after treatment with veratrine, barium and guanidine, *Chin. J. Physiol.,* 16, 143, 1941.

7. **Riker, W. F., Jr., Roberts, J., Standaert, F. G., and Fujimori, H.,** The motor nerve terminal as the primary focus for drug-induced facilitation of neuromuscular transmission, *J. Pharmacol. Exp. Ther.,* 121, 286, 1957.

8. **Standaert, F. G.,** Post-tetanic activity in the cat soleus nerve; its origin, course and mechanism of generation, *J. Gen. Physiol.,* 47, 53, 1963.

9. **Standaert, F. G.,** The mechanisms of post-tetanic potentiation in cat soleus and gastrocnemius muscles, *J. Gen. Physiol.,* 47, 987, 1964.

10. **Burke, R. E.,** Motor units: anatomy, physiology and functional organization, in *Handbook of Physiology, Section 1, The Nervous System,* Vol. II. *Motor Control, Part 1,* Brookhart, J. M., Mountcastte, V. B., Brooks, V. B., and Geiger, S. R., Ed., American Physiological Society, Bethesda, 1982, 345.

11. **Storella, R. J., Riker, W. F., Jr., and Baker, T.,** Effects of adrenalectomy on neostigmine-induced facilitation on mammalian motor nerve terminal function, *Fed. Proc.,* 40, 262, 1981.

12. **Baker, T. and Dorato, A.,** Pharmacologic differences between rat tonic and phasic motor nerve terminals, *Fed. Proc.,* 40, 261, 1981.

13. **Baker, T. and Stanec, A.,** A prejunction effect of neostigmine on terminals of phasic and tonic motor nerves in adult and aged rats. *Anesthesiology,* Suppl. 59, A281, 1982.

14. **Lowndes, H. E., Baker, T., and Riker, W. F., Jr.,** Motor nerve dysfunction in delayed DFP neuropathy, *Eur. J. Pharmacol.,* 29, 66, 1974.

15. **Cavanagh, J. B.,** The significance of the dying back process in experimental and human neurological disease, *Int. Rev. Exp. Pathol.,* 3, 219, 1964.

16. **Lowndes, H. E. and Baker, T.,** Studies on drug-induced neuropathies. III. Motor nerve deficit in cats with experimental acrylamide neuropathy, *Eur. J. Pharmacol.,* 35, 177, 1976.

17. **Spencer, P. S. and Schaumburg, H. H.,** Ultrastructural studies of the dying-back process. III. The evolution of experimental peripheral giant axonal degeneration, *J. Neuropathol. Exp. Neurol.,* 36, 276, 1977.

18. **Baker, T., Lowndes, H. E., Johnson, M. K., and Sandborg, I. C.,** The effects of phenylmethansulfonyl fluoride on delayed organophosphorus neuropathy, *Arch. Toxicol.,* 46, 305, 1980.

19. **Baker, T., Drakontides, A. B. and Riker, W. F., Jr.,** Prevention of the organophosphorus neuropathy by glucocorticoids, *Exp. Neurol.,* 78, 197, 1982.

20. **Drakontides, A. B. and Baker, T.,** An electrophysiologic and ultrastructural study of the phenylmethane-sulfonyl fluoride protection against a delayed organophosphorus neuropathy, *Toxicol. Appl. Pharmacol.,* 70, 411, 1983.

21. **Lowndes, H. E., Baker, T., and Riker, W. F., Jr.,** Motor nerve terminal response to edrophonium in delayed DFP neuropathy, *Eur. J. Pharmacol.,* 30, 69, 1975.

22. **Howland, R. D., Lowndes, H. E., Baker, T., and Richardson, R. J.,** DFP mononeuropathy: evidence for a peripheral site of initiation, *Brain Res.,* 1184, 248, 1980.

23. **Glazer, E. F., Baker, T., and Riker, W. F., Jr.,** The neuropathology of DFP at cat soleus neuromuscular junction, *J. Neurocytol.,* 7, 741, 1978.

24. **Drakontides, A. B., Baker, T., and Riker, W. F., Jr.,** A morphological study of the effect of gluco-corticoid treatment on delayed organophosphorus neuropathy, *Neurotoxicology,* 3(4), 165, 1982.

25. **Baker, T., Glazer, E., and Lowndes, H. E.,** Subacute neuropathic effects of diisopropylfluorophosphate at the cat soleus neuromuscular junction, *Neuropathol. Appl. Neurobiol.,* 3, 377, 1977.

26. **Baker, T. and Stanec, A.,** Methylprednisolone treatment of an organophosphorus-induced delayed neu-ropathy, *Toxicol. Appl. Pharmacol.,* 79, 348, 1985.

27. **Lowndes, H. E. and Baker, T.,** Toxic site of action in distal axonopathies, in *Experimental and Clinical Neurotoxicology,* Spencer, P. S. and Schaumburg, H. H., Ed., Williams & Wilkins, Baltimore, 1980, 193.

28. **Lowndes, H. E., Baker, T., Cho, S. E., and Jortner, B. S.,** Position sensitivity of de-efferented muscle spindles in experimental acrylamide neuropathy, *J. Pharmacol. Exp. Ther.,* 205, 40, 1978.

29. **Lowndes, H. E., Baker, T., Michelson, L. P., and Vincent-Ablazey, M.,** Attenuated dynamic responses of primary endings of muscle spindles: a basis for depressed tendon responses in acrylamide neuropathy, *Ann. Neurol.,* 3, 433, 1978.

30. **Goldstein, B. D., Lowndes, H. E., and Cho, E. S.,** Neurotoxicology of vincristine in the cat: electro-physiological studies, *Arch. Toxicol.,* 48, 253, 1981.

31. **Cho, E. S., Lowndes, H. E., and Goldstein, B. D.,** Neurotoxicology of vincristine in the cat: morphological study, *Arch. Toxicol.,* 52, 83, 1983.

32. **Baker, T. and Lowndes, H. E.,** The effect of iminodipropiontrile on mammalian motor nerve endings, *Pharmacologist,* 26, 230, 1984.

Chapter 10

SYNAPTIC TOXICOLOGY OF ENVIRONMENTAL AGENTS

George G. Bierkamper

I.   Introduction 104

II.   Metals 105
     A.   Lead...105
     B.   Mercury 109
     C.   Organotin Compounds...114

III.   Insecticides 115
     A.   Pyrethroids 115
     B.   Halogenated Hydrocarbons 117
     C.   Lindane 119
     D.   DDT..120
     E.   Anticholinesterase Agents 121

V.   Other Neurotoxic Compounds 125
     A.   Dithiobiuret 125
     B.   Aliphatic Alcohols...126
     C.   2,5 Hexanedione 129

IV.   Conclusions...131

Acknowledgments 133

References..133

I. INTRODUCTION

This chapter reviews synaptic toxicology as viewed through the oscilloscope, i.e., as examined by electrophysiological methods. Numerous drugs, natural toxins, and chemical compounds alter synaptic function; however, it is the aim of this chapter to focus on selected chemicals which concern the environmental toxicologist. Within this criterion, we will examine a small, but growing literature in which electrophysiological techniques have been employed for the purpose of *elucidating the mechanism of action of neurotoxic substances.* As a consequence, numerous studies whose focus is general synaptic physiology and pharmacology will not be included even though they represent, in many cases, important contributions to our understanding of synaptic malfunction and malleability.

The mammalian synapse is the electrophysical gap across which a neuronal signal must traverse via chemical mediation. Synapses connect neurons to neurons or neurons to neuroeffector cells and provide fine control of signal transmission throughout the body in much the same way it relays operate in telephone networks. Interruption of neurohumoral transmission at the synapse effectively stops meaningful signal transfer and thus distinguishes this as a vulnerable target of neurotoxic insult.

Since neurotransmission across the synapse is a complex series of electrical events (as described in detail in Chapter 3), it is most useful to study synaptic toxicology with electrophysiological techniques such as intracellular recording. These techniques have advantages over other methods, e.g., histology, by virtue of their ability to analyze realtime events at the synapse in a dynamic state of function rather than at a frozen point in time. Nonetheless, they have intrinsic technical and interpretative limitations as the complexity of nervous system increases. Consequently, the majority of reports in the literature employ electrophysiological methods to study synaptic toxicology in relatively simple systems such as the neuromuscular junction. It can be argued, nevertheless, that the toxicological information gathered at this synapse may be, in principle, readily extrapolated to CNS synapses. Thus, the neuromuscular junction will serve as a model synapse for most of the discussions in this chapter.

Toxic manifestations at the neuromuscular junction and other synapses are expressed as an interference of normal signal transmission and include a wide range of effects from the most subtle deficiencies in neurotransmitter release to complete block of transmission and ultrastructural disintegration of the synapse. The target of toxicity may be either a presynaptic or a postsynaptic element or both. Presynaptically, a toxic insult will interfere with neurotransmission in the simplest terms by altering transmitter release. There are a large number of vulnerable elements in the nerve terminal that can contribute to changes in transmitter release if compromised by a toxic compound. In general, these include (1) transmitter synthesis and/or packaging, (2) delivery of axonally transported materials to the nerve terminal, (3) the release mechanism(s), (4) structural integrity of the terminal, (5) bioenergetic systems, and (6) biomembrane processes related to excitability and maintenance of the membrane potential.

Postsynaptically, the primary element of neurotransmission is the specific receptor upon which the transmitter acts to signal the postsynaptic cell. A toxic insult in this region will thus effect (1) the reception of released neurotransmitter, (2) the removal or elimination of neurotransmitter from the reception area, or (3) the transduction of the neurotransmitter-receptor interaction.

The present review will examine the literature on the synaptic toxicology of lead, mercury, triethyltin, pyrethroids, halogenated hydrocarbon insecticides, anticholinesterase agents, dithiobiuret, aliphatic alcohols, 2,5-hexanedione, and the actions and interactions of other selected compounds. In addition, the present review aims to demonstrate how electrophysiological methods have been used to determine whether the neurotoxic mechanism of a compound is pre- or postsynaptic or, both. Further, it is of interest to determine how far these methods can go in actually resolving an intraterminal toxic mechanism such as mitochondrial damage. In this regard, the advantages and shortcomings of the electrophysiological techniques will become apparent.

II. METALS

A. Lead

Lead is a major element of environmental concern (e.g., leaded gasoline) and has been the focus of intense research and controversy in recent years. Kostial and Vouk[61] demonstrated blockade of ganglionic transmission in perfused superior cervical ganglia of cats by lead nitrate in concentrations as low as 12 μM. They deduced that the decreased contractions of the nictitating membrane were due to a presynaptic effect of lead ions whereby calcium-dependent acetylcholine (ACh) output was reduced. The classic paper of Manalis and Cooper[70] was the first to employ electrophysiological techniques to the study of the effect of lead on neuromuscular transmission. Using intracellular recording techniques in the frog sciatic nerve-sartorius muscle preparation, these authors discovered that Pb^{2+} increased miniature end-plate potentials (MEPP) frequency and depressed endplate potential (EPP) amplitude in a dose-dependent manner. These effects were reversible by washing lead out of the preparation. The dose and temporal differential between the increase in MEPP frequency and the decrease in facilitated EPP amplitudes provoked speculation that these two processes were distinct, but not entirely independent. Iontophoretic application of ACh to the endplate ruled out a significant postjunctional effect of lead (0.10 mM). The authors concluded that lead had a predominantly presynaptic action and that it was similar to other divalent cations (Ln, Mg, Be, Mn, Ni, and Zn) in its ability to inhibit the phasic release of transmitter.

A decade later, Cooper and Manalis[28-30] resumed their studies on the synaptic action of lead. Since the effect of Pb^{2+} on phasic transmitter release was readily reversible and with the demonstration that Pb^{2+} blocked the uptake of Ca^{2+} into the nerve terminals of the frog sympathetic ganglion,[57] it was argued that a competitive interaction existed between Pb^{2+} and Ca^{2+}. This was experimentally established by comparing dose-response curves of EPP amplitudes vs. calcium concentration in the absence and presence of 1 μM Pb^{2+} (Figure 1A). The parallel shift to the right of the log-log plots strengthened the argument, and eliminated the concern, that the altered ionic medium (low Ca^{2+}; high Mg^{2+}) required for twitch-free intracellular recording, distorted the results. Further proof of a competitive interaction between Pb^{2+} and Ca^{2+} was presented in an unusual modified Lineweaver-Burke plot of the reciprocal of the fifth root of the EPP against the reciprocal of the Ca^{2+} concentration (Figure 1B). The similarity of the y-intercepts indicated competitive antagonism by Pb^{2+} assuming the nth root of the EPP amplitude is correctly 5.[28,33]

In contrast to this extracellular competition, an hypothesis was presented that lead acts intracellularly to raise MEPP frequency. This was supported by the time delay between the decrease in EPP amplitude and the increase in MEPP frequency, presumably due to the time required for Pb^{2+} to enter the cell. These results were recently corroborated by examining the interactive effects of cadmium and Pb^{2+} on evoked and spontaneous transmitter release in the frog muscle preparation (Figure 2).[29] It was concluded that Pb^{2+} and Cd^{2+} compete with Ca^{2+} for a common presynaptic recognition site during evoked transmitter release. Cd^{2+} also appeared to inhibit the entry of Pb^{2+} into the nerve terminal where it may act to induce an increase in spontaneous transmitter release (Figure 3). The incompletely arithmatical additive effects of Cd^{2+} and Pb^{2+} along with similar comparisons by these and other investigators has culminated in an intriguing theoretical dissertation by Cooper and colleagues[31] on the effects of polyvalent cations on transmitter release as a consequence of the ionic radius and hydration energy.

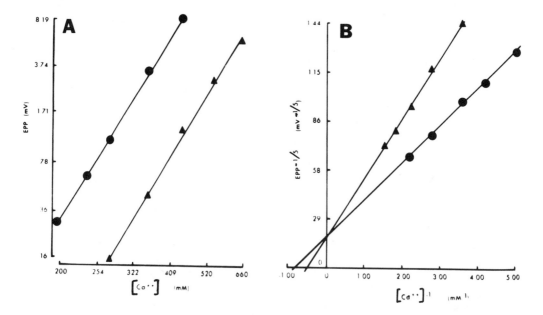

FIGURE 1 A and B.   Reduction of evoked ACh release by Pb^{++} through competitive interaction with Ca^{++} at frog neuromuscular junction. The same data were plotted in two different ways to demonstrate the relationship between $[Ca^{++}]$ in the Ringer solution and the average amplitude of the EPP obtained first in the absence of (solid circles) and then in the presence of (solid triangles) 1 μM Pb^{++}. (A) Data plotted on log-log coordinates. Pb^{++} shifted the relationship to the right with no change in slope. (B) Modified Lineweaver-Burke plots of the reciprocal of the fifth root of the EPP against the reciprocal of $[Ca^{++}]$. The competitive interaction of Pb^{++} is shown by similarity of the y-intercepts (0.162 for control and 0.157 for Pb^{++} by regression analysis). Each point represents the average of 200 EPPs; the nerve was stimulated at 0.5 Hz; $[Mg^{++}] = 2.9$ mM. (From Manalis, R. S. et al., *Brain Res.*, 294, 95, 1984. With permission.)

In vitro effects of lead have also been studied electrophysiologically at the mammalian neuromuscular junction by Atchison and Narahashi.[12] Evoked and spontaneous transmitter release were examined by conventional intracellular recording techniques in the rat hemi-diaphragm preparation (Figure 4). Nerve-evoked release (EPP) was rapidly depressed by 25 and 52% by lead acetate at 20 and 100 μM, respectively. These results are not unlike the effects of lead at the frog neuromuscular junction except that the rat neuromuscular junction requires higher concentrations of lead to block the EPP. Lead (100 μM) increased MEPP frequency by approximately four to five times control values in agreement with the findings at frog neuromuscular junction. This study extends the previous work at the neuromuscular junction by more completely applying the power of intracellular recording methods through the calculation of the statistical parameters of transmitter release. Despite the interpretative shortcomings of these calculations (see Chapter 3) they can direct one's attention, at least grossly, to the possible location of neurotoxic insult within the neurotransmitter release pathway of the nerve terminal. For example, Atchison and Narahashi observed that mean quantal content (m) was reduced in the presence of lead and could be accounted for primarily by a decrease in the immediately releasable store of transmitter (n) as calculated by $n = m/p$. The probability of transmitter release (p) was estimated from the mean and variance of the MEPP's and EPP's and was unchanged or slightly increased by the lead treatment. Although not clearly understood, the parameter n is thought to represent the site through which Ca^{2+} is linked to stimulus secretion. The observed decrease in n strengthened their argument that lead interferes competitively with Ca^{2+} at the membrane entry level where Ca^{2+} normally triggers the release of prepackaged transmitter.

Atchison and Narahashi[12] also found that extracellular Ca^{2+} was unnecessary for lead to

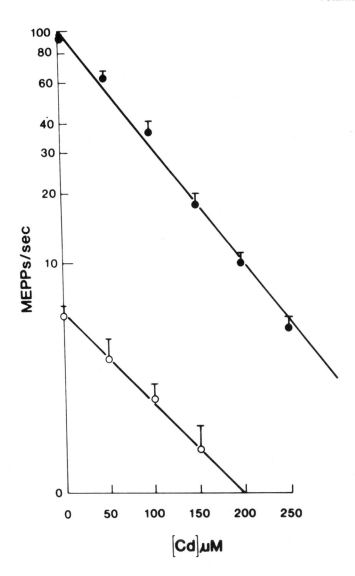

FIGURE 2. Effects of Cd^{++} on Pb^{++}-induced increases in MEPP frequency. Two separate experiments are shown. $[Pb^{++}]$ was maintained at 50 μM. Each experiment began with the highest concentration of Cd^{++} (250 or 150 μM). MEPP frequency was measured with successively lower concentrations allowing 10 min between solution changes. The log of MEPP frequency is plotted against $[Cd^{++}]$. Values represent mean ± standard deviation. Linear regression analysis of the data yields r = 0.97 for solid circles and r = 0.99 for open circles. $[Ca^{++}] = 0.5$ m*M* and $[Mg^{++}] = 6.0$ m*M*. (From Cooper, G. P. and Manalis, R. S., *Neurotoxicology*, 4, 69, 1983. With permission.)

increase MEPP frequency. In concert with Cooper and Manalis, they concluded that lead must enter the cell in order to stimulate spontaneous release; consequently, they speculated that lead increases cytoplasmic Ca^{2+} by interfering with the complex Ca^{2+}-buffering processes within the nerve terminal. This is supported by the study of Kolton and Yaari[58] concerning the effects of in vitro lead on intraneuronal Ca^{2+} in the frog sartorius preparation. Furthermore, other substances (e.g., ruthenium red) which interfere with Ca^{2+} sequestration in the nerve terminal also increase MEPP frequency.[90]

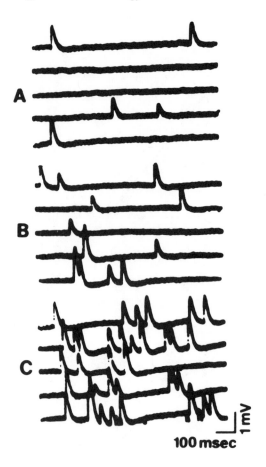

FIGURE 3. Incomplete antagonism of Pb^{++}-induced increases in MEPP frequency by Cd^{++}. (A) Control MEPP frequency; (B) MEPP frequency in the presence of 50 μM Pb^{++} and 100 μM Cd^{++} demonstrating the partial block by Cd^{++} of the Pb^{++}-induced increase in MEPP frequency; and (C) MEPP frequency in the presence of 50 μM Pb^{++}. [Ca^{++}] = 0.4 mM and [Mg^{++}] = 5.0 mM throughout the experiment. (From Cooper, G. P. and Manalis, R. S., *Toxicol. Appl. Phamarcol.*, 74, 411, 1984. With permission.)

In 1984, Manalis and co-workers published a thorough electrophysiological study on the in vitro effect of lead at the frog neuromuscular junction. Although largely repetitive of their previous studies, this work is a more rigorous investigation of the competitive interactions of Ca^{2+} and Pb^{2+} on neuromuscular transmission. Unlike Atchison and Narahashi who found no change in MEPP amplitude, Manalis and co-workers observed that MEPP amplitude decreased transiently when MEPP frequency was increased by lead. At a constant dose of Pb^{2+} (50 μM) the increase in MEPP frequency reached a peak at about 2.5 min then declined exponentially towards control levels. Lead did not alter the input resistance of muscle fibers nor did it significantly effect the postjunctional potential of iontophoretically applied ACh when localized at the end-plate. Technically difficult extracellular recordings from the nerve terminal revealed no interruption of the terminal potential (depolarization). Lead was determined to be 3 × 10^3 times more potent than Mg^{2+} in antagonizing the Ca^{2+} receptive site (dissociation constant of Pb^{2+} at this site equals 0.99 μM) and thus blocking ACh

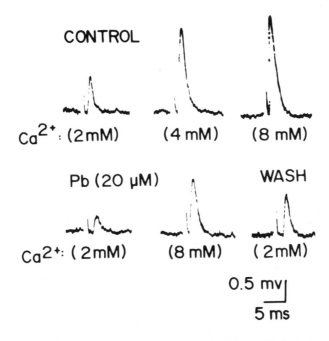

FIGURE 4.   Effects of increasing bath [Ca^{++}] on EPP amplitudes before and after treatment with 100 μM Pb^{++}. EPPs are taken from the same end-plate of a representative preparation. *d*-Tubocurarine was present to prevent muscular contraction during nerve stimulation. (From Atchison, W. D. and Narahashi, T., *Neurotoxicology*, 5, 267, 1984. With permission.)

release. Furthermore, Pb was three times more potent than Cd^{2+} and about 150 times more potent than Mn^{2+} or Co^{2+} in blocking this site. These authors concluded that lead may effect evoked transmitter release by (1) interfering with Ca^{2+} entry through voltage-sensitive Ca^{2+} channels during depolarization of the nerve terminal rather than (2) via the interaction of Ca^{2+} with the synaptic vesicles and the active zones to induce exocytosis. Atchison and Narahashi[12] interpreted their results to favor the interaction of Pb^{2+} with the latter mechanism. However, the uncertainty of the significance of the statistical parameter *n* and the persuasive arguments in the Manalis et al.[72] study strongly suggest the interaction of Pb^{2+} at the voltage-dependent Ca^{2+} membrane site.

It is disappointing that all the electrophysiological studies on the synaptic toxicity of lead have been confined to in vitro exposure with the exception of Audesirk and Audesirk.[16] Chronic low-level lead exposure (5 μM) in the freshwater pond snail *Lymnaea stagnalis* induced significant alterations in the neuronal physiology of individually identifiable neurons in isolated brain.[16] Lead increased resting membrane potential of most neuron types, delayed the recovery of the spike undershoot, decreased input resistance, and decreased spontaneous spiking activity. Although synaptic transmission was not directly assessed, one would predict flawed signal transfer by virtue of the observed changes in neuronal excitability. How this chronic study and the previous in vitro studies relate to the neurotoxicity of chronic low-level lead exposure to mammals is uncertain. There is clearly a compelling need to conduct further electrophysiological experiments on the in vivo effects of lead on synaptic transmission.

B. Mercury

The toxic effects of inorganic and organic mercury on synaptic transmission have been examined by electrophysiological techniques in only a few reports over the past decade. Manalis and Cooper[71] observed a phasic potentiation of EPP amplitude by 1.0 μM HgCl$_2$

in the isolated frog sartorius preparation. Mean EPP amplitude increased from 1.4 mV control to a peak of 7.3 mV within 35 min, then irreversibly declined to 0 after 1 hr. MEPP frequency was unaffected by 1.0 μM Hg^{2+} or lower, but was increased at concentrations of 10 μM or more. Local iontophoretic application of ACh to the end-plate demonstrated the lack of a postsynaptic effect in vitro Hg^{2+} (1.0 and 10.0 μM). The authors concluded that the massive increase in EPP amplitude was due to a prejunctional effect of Hg^{2+} and introduced the intriguing hypothesis that Hg^{2+} bridges sulfhydryl sites normally associated with Ca^{2+}-evoked release of transmitter. The initial effects of Hg^{2+} on evoked release, therefore, differ from those observed for Pb^{2+} in two ways: (1) EPP amplitude increased dramatically prior to block and (2) the increase in MEPP frequency at a relatively high dose of Hg^{2+} (10 μM) occurred simultaneously with the block in evoked release, perhaps revealing rapid intracellular penetration of Hg^{2+}.[23]

Juang[50] presented a detailed electrophysiological report on the in vitro actions of methylmercuric chloride and mercuric chloride on frog sciatic nerve-sartorius muscle. HgCl$_2$ (0.04 mM), but not CH$_3$HgCl (0.04 mM), depolarized the resting membrane potential and depressed the effective myofiber resistance and action potential amplitude. Muscle fibers eventually became electrically inexcitable. Both compounds induced large, transient increases in MEPP frequency and evoked transmitter release then caused complete suppression of transmitter release within 10 to 15 min. The author speculated that both compounds share a common prejunctional site of action and provided a thorough discussion of the possibilities, including sulfhydryl binding and cationic interactions.

Miyamoto[76] further probed the mechanism of in vitro neurotoxicity of Hg^{2+} in a recent study employing intracellular recording techniques in the frog cutaneous pectoris muscle preparation. This work confirmed the earlier study of Manalis and Cooper[71] showing that Hg^{2+} transiently increases transmitter release, then irreversibly blocks transmitter release (EPPs). In addition, Hg^{2+} (3 μM) transiently increased MEPP frequency in partially K$^+$-depolarized preparations then caused the disappearance of MEPPs with no obvious effect on the postsynaptic receptors. It was argued that the MEPP discharge is blocked by Hg^{2+}-induced depolarization of the nerve terminals. Miyamoto next tested the hypothesis that the initial increase in transmitter release by Hg^{2+} may be due to entry of ionic mercury through ionic channels where its intraterminal presence would promote transmitter release.[24] He recorded MEPPs in the presence of Co^{2+} (a Ca channel antagonist) and Hg^{2+} to determine if ionic mercury enters the nerve terminal through Ca channels only and in the presence of tetrodotoxin (TTX, a Na channel blocker) to test for Na channel entry. Neither Co^{2+} or TTX alone blocked the Hg^{2+}-induced increase in MEPP frequency. However, when used in combination, the two channel blockers prevented the increase in MEPP frequency associated with Hg^{2+} (Figure 5). This is a very interesting discovery suggesting that Hg^{2+} exerts its neurotoxic effect at an intracellular site by gaining access through both Na and Ca channels. This apparently applies only to inorganic mercury since this study shows a lower dose effectiveness of CH$_3$Hg$^+$ (100 μM) in order to mimic the responses of Hg^{2+} (3 μM), and a failure of TTX and Co^{2+} to block the enhancement by methylmercury of MEPP frequency. It is likely that methylmercury readily penetrates the nerve terminal membrane by virtue of its high lipid solubility.

The effects of Hg^{2+} on neurotransmitter release are postulated to involve the extremely high affinity of Hg^{2+} for SH groups at the level of the release mechanism (screening of internal negative charges or binding of the synaptic vesicles to the nerve terminal membrane[76]). Sulfhydryl reagents are also known to interact with SH groups on the ACh nicotinic receptor producing changes in end-plate current time constants.[102] With the evidence of presynaptic cholinoceptors regulating ACh release from motorneurons[19,73,117] and CNS nerve endings it seems pertinent to reexamine the effects of Hg^{2+} on the modulatory mechanisms of neurotransmitter release.[37]

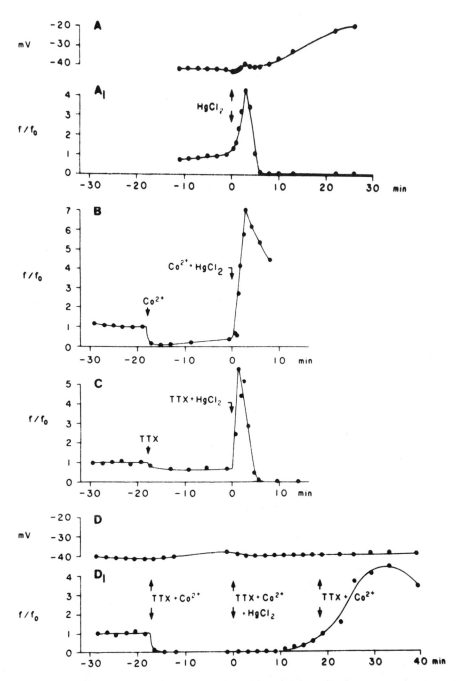

FIGURE 5.   Effect of channel blocking agents on the response to Hg^{++} in a frog neuromuscular preparation. Panels A (muscle membrane potential) and A_1 (MEPP frequency) show control responses to 3 μM $HgCl_2$. For comparative purposes, frequencies (f) are normalized to fractions (f/f$_o$) of the frequency immediately before the application of $HgCl_2$ (f$_o$). In all cases onset of $HgCl_2$ is indicated by time 0. Note the marked depolarization and rapid rise and then fall in MEPP frequency. Panel B shows the MEPP frequency response to 3 μM $HgCl_2$ following pretreatment with and in the presence of 1.8 mM Co^{++} alone. Panel C shows the same experiment using 3.13 μM TTX alone. Neither agent alone blocked the Hg^{++}-induced alteration of MEPP frequency. Panels D and D_1 represent the responses to 3 μM $HgCl_2$ following pretreatment with and in the presence of both blocking agents, 3.13 μM TTX and 1.8 mM Co^{++} (Co^{++} was substituted for Ca^{++} to avoid changing the divalent cation concentration). Note that both membrane depolarization and the effect on MEPP frequency are blocked. The block of the frequency increase was gradually overcome (t = 10 min). (From Miyamoto, M. D., *Brain Res.*, 267, 375, 1983. With permission.)

Binah and colleagues[23] pursued the hypothesis that the effects the inorganic mercurial, $HgCl_2$, and the mercurial, mersalyl, on neurotransmitter release are correlated to a subcellular mechanism (e.g., mitochondrial calcium transport) regulating intraterminal Ca^+ concentrations. Verifying the work above, they found that Hg^{2+} (0.5 μM) and mersalyl (5 μM) increased, then later decreased both the spontaneous and evoked transmitter release as measured by intracellular recordings in the frog sartorius preparation. These concentrations of mercury were found to inhibit mitochondrial calcium transport as well as calcium transport in isolated synaptosomal vesicles. Since mitochondrial oxidative phosphorylation was not impaired by these concentrations of mercury, it was concluded that the increase in MEPP frequency and EPP amplitude was a direct consequence of the intraterminal increase in Ca^{2+} when mitochondrial and vesicular calcium transport was inhibited. To explain the later depression in neurotransmitter release, these investigators suggested that increases in intraterminal mercury levels are likely to disrupt other mechanisms involving $-SH$ groups. It is prudent to assume that these latter effects of mercury are of greater significance to the chronically exposed human nervous system.

Barrett et al.[17a] presented a revealing preliminary study on the irreversible blocking action of methylmercury (1 to 3 ppm) on neuromuscular transmission in frog cutaneous pectoris muscle. Methylmercury (10 ppm) increased MEPP frequency 100 to 1000 times above control rates and subsequently blocked neurotransmission. Extracellular recording from the nerve terminal nerve branches demonstrated a disappearance of nerve action potentials. The authors concluded that methylmercury causes a failure of the presynaptic nerve action potential to propagate at the nerve terminal, thus blocking transmission.

Atchison and Narahashi[11] published a detailed study of the in vitro effects of micromolar concentrations of methylmercury on neurotransmission in the isolated rat phrenic nerve-hemidiaphragm using intracellular recording methods. In brief, MEPP frequency was increased by 20 and 100 μM methylmercury, the effects occurring more rapidly with the higher dose (Figure 6) in agreement with earlier studies.[50,51] MEPP amplitude and resting membrane potential were unaffected. Under conditions of high Mg^{2+} and low Ca^{2+}, EPP amplitude was decreased and finally blocked by 20 and 100 μM of methylmercury, but not by 4 μM (Figure 6). Intermittent iontophoretic application of ACh produced end-plate depolarizations which did not vary even after 30 min of 100 μM methylmercury exposure, thus eliminating the possible contribution of the postjunctional receptor alterations. Determination of the statistical parameters of release revealed a decrease in quantal content (m), a significant increase in the probability of release (p), and a decrease in the immediately available store (n) as measured 15 min after the introduction of 20 μM methylmercury. The parameters of release were not different from control with 4 μM methylmercury and could not be calculated at 100 μM due to the rapid, irreversible block of the EPPs. Atchison and Narahashi speculated, based primarily on the observed increase in p, that the molecular mechanism of methylmercury in altering neurotransmitter release is linked to Ca^{2+} movement across the cell membrane via channels or to intraterminal Ca^{2+} mismanagement. This theory seems plausible because of the similarity of the results with other polyvalent cations (Co^{2+}, Mn^{2+}, and La^{3+}) suspected to be Ca channel blockers.[31] Further support for this theory has been demonstrated by Alkadhi and Taha[5a] in the superior cervical ganglion of the rabbit where increases in extracellular Ca^{2+} antagonized the inhibitory effects of methylmercury on ganglionic transmission.

A more thorough discussion of the presynaptic effects of methylmercury may be found in a recent review by Atchison and co-workers[13] which reiterates the results described above. In addition, this study reports the use of La^{3+} to reverse the late depression in MEPP frequency caused by 100 μM methylmercury, thus providing evidence that transmitter stores were not depleted (Figure 7).[13] Moreover, electron micrographs of methylmercury-poisoned mouse neuromuscular junctions revealed normal end-plate ultrastructure with a full com-

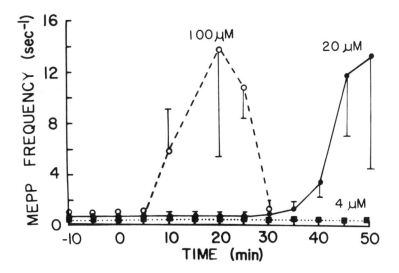

FIGURE 6. Time course of the effects on methylmercury on MEPP frequency in a rat phrenic nerve-hemidiaphragm preparation. MEPPs were recorded continuously for 10 min before and up to 50 min after 4, 20, or 100 μM methylmercury introduced at time 0. Values represent the mean ± SEM of 3 to 8 determinations. MEPP frequency was determined over 5 min increments. (From Atchison, W. D. and Narahashi, T., *Neurotoxicology,* 3, 37, 1982. With permission.)

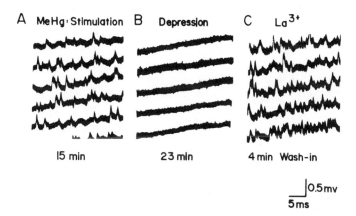

FIGURE 7. Effects of lanthanum (La^{+++}) on late depression of MEPP frequency induced by methylmercury (100 μM). Mepps were recorded from the same cell during increased MEPP frequency (A), and decreased MEPP frequency (B) following methylmercury. When no further MEPPs were recorded, 100 μM methylmercury and 1 mM $LaCl_3$ were introduced (C). (From Atchison, W. D. et al., *Cellular and Molecular Neurotoxicology,* Raven Press, New York, 1984. With permission.)

plement of synaptic vesicles, even though the functional correlate at the time of fixation showed MEPP frequency decreasing.[13] It is clear, therefore, that in vitro methylmercury has predominantly a presynaptic action on the ACh release mechanism.

The in vitro effects of methylmercury on synaptic transmission differ from other polyvalent cations in that (1) they are irreversible and (2) they cause a late cessation of spontaneous release of neurotransmitter. Nonetheless, it is uncertain how the results of these in vitro studies apply to the neuromuscular and CNS disorders associated with chronic mercury poisoning.

C. Organotin Compounds

Triethyltin (TET) is a potent neurotoxicant whose manifestations of neuromuscular weakness have been traced, in part, to depression of neurotransmission.[20] Like most of the literature searches on the synaptic toxicity of selected neurotoxic compounds, one finds several earlier reports on muscle twitch,[17,105] but only one where the effects of TET on synaptic transmission were studied by electrophysiological methods.[6] Allen and co-workers studied the in vitro effects of TET in the mouse sternomastoid muscle using intracellular microelectrodes. TET sulfate (10^{-7} to 10^{-5} M) induced a dose-dependent decrease in EPP amplitude, but had no effect on MEPP amplitude, indicating a presynaptic rather than postsynaptic action. This site of action had been previously suggested by muscle contraction studies.[17] The reduction in EPP amplitude to 20% of control by TET (5×10^{-6} M) for 70 min was not reversible by attempted washout with normal buffered medium. Since spontaneous release was unaffected, the authors argued that TET did not effect the release mechanism per se, but rather it may interfere with calcium conduction across the terminal membrane. However, no evidence was presented to support this theory. Bierkamper and co-workers[121] tested adult male rats exposed to TET bromide (30 mg/ℓ) in their drinking water for 1, 2, or 3 weeks, then examined neuromuscular transmission in the isolated cut phrenic nerve-hemidiaphragm preparation. Resting membrane potential in the cut preparation drops to approximately -45mV so that subtle toxicant-induced changes in resting membrane potential (RMP) cannot be detected; however, cutting prevents muscular contraction and allows nerve activity to be studied without the use of twitch prevention treatments, i.e., curare or low Ca, high Mg. Preliminary experiments indicated MEPP activity and low-frequency (0.1 to 1 Hz) EPPs were within normal limits in the hemidiaphragms from subchronically treated TET subjects. However, EPP amplitudes decreased rapidly when tetanic stimulation (40 Hz) was applied to the phrenic nerve (2- and 3-week treatment groups), revealing deficiencies in the capacity of the nerve to release ACh under demanding conditions. This deficiency in stimulated ACh release was verified by direct biochemical measurement of endogenous ACh efflux from phrenic nerve-hemidiaphragm preparation isolated from TET-treated rats.[22] Most interesting, in terms of the mechanism of action of TET, was the preliminary observation of a greatly prolonged elevation of post-stimulus MEPP frequency following a 2-sec burst of 150 to 200 Hz nerve stimulation.[122] This prolonged elevation in MEPP frequency resembled the action of ruthenium red, which is known to block Ca^{2+} uptake into mitochondria.[40,90] Thus, together with the evidence that TET is a mitochondrial poison,[5,77,80] it is postulated that TET induces intraterminal Ca^{2+} mismanagement by interfering with mitochondrial uptake of Ca^{2+} during higher frequencies of stimulation, leading to an enhancement of spontaneous release.[90] In this regard, subchronic TET treatment appears to provoke an effect in the driven isolated preparations similar to in vitro Hg^{2+} intoxication.[71]

In situ intracellular recording from soleus muscle of rats revealed a decrease in RMP in vivo with subchronic TET exposure.[75] The consistent presence of spontaneous MEPP activity and the rapid recovery of RMP after TET was withdrawn eliminated denervation as the possible cause of TET-induced depolarization of the muscle membranes.[101]

Although TET undoubtedly alters mitochondrial function, its primary action may be on excitable cell membranes as well as mitochondrial membranes.[103] A number of studies report that TET alters membrane permeability, particularly to Cl^-.[20,96,107,115] These observations distinguish TET from other metabolic neurotoxic compounds studied and demonstrate the usefulness of continued studies on TET as a model compound which effects anionic membrane conductances by an ionophoric carrier mechanism without interfering with an existing anion channel. This action would appear to differ from the action of Hg^{2+}, Pb^{2+}, or other polyvalent cations that are usually associated with competitive antagonism of Ca^{2+} at the level of a membrane channel or receptive site linked to the neurotransmitter release process.[31]

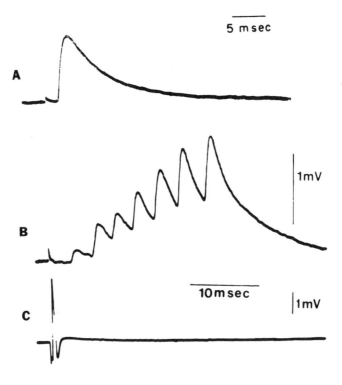

FIGURE 8.   Effects of allethrin on neuromuscular transmission. Normal EPPs recorded in frog sciatic nerve-sartorius preparation (A). Repetitive EPPs (B) and action potential of the sciatic nerve (C) recorded simultaneously on stimulation of the ventral spinal root after 50 min of exposure to 1 μM allethrin. Note the absence of repetitive activity in the sciatic nerve. (From Wouters, W. et al., *Eur. J. Pharmacol.*, 43, 163, 1977. With permission).

III. INSECTICIDES

A. Pyrethroids

Pyrethroid insecticides, including natural pyrethrins, are known to alter nervous system function in many organisms.[98,120] The neurotoxic effects of the pyrethroid, allethrin, have been explored by an exceptionally adept use of electrophysiological techniques in frog motor neurons and end-plates.[108,119] In the presence of allethrin (as low as 10^{-7} M) a single nerve impulse was observed to elicit up to 13 end-plate potentials as measured by intracellular microelectrodes (Figure 8). The repetitive activity showed an inverse temperature dependence and was not associated with proximal nerve firing or backfiring. Indeed, the repetitive discharges were confined to the nerve terminal region. This was demonstrated by delicate extracellular recording along the motor neurons and terminal branches. Additional experiments were performed in which the sciatic nerve was dissected free to the level of the Xth spinal nerve with intact ventral and dorsal roots. Allethrin induced marked repetitive activity in the dorsal spinal root (sensory) when a brief stimulus was applied to the sciatic nerve, but did not evoke repetitive activity in the ventral spinal root (motor) nor did the motor neurons exhibit repetitive firing. Only at the end-plate did stimulation of the ventral roots cause repetitive activity. Consequently, the authors state that it is unlikely that the repetitive activity is similar to that observed in the presence of acetylcholinesterase inhibitors.[1,2,53] Allethrin did not alter MEPP frequency or amplitude even at the concentration of 10^{-5} M in vitro for 2 hr. Initial EPP amplitude and time course were unaltered; however, the repetitive

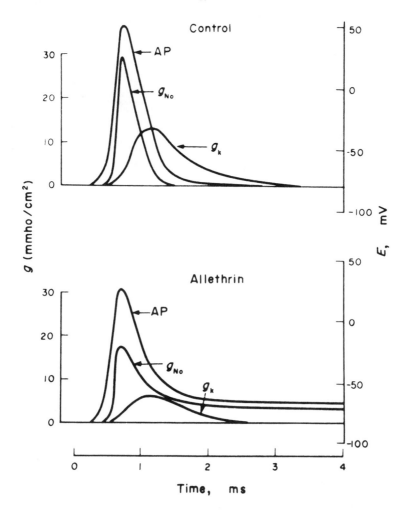

FIGURE 9.   Diagram of the time courses of the action potential (AP), the membrane conductance (g_{Na}), and the membrane potassium conductance (g_K) before and during the application of allethrin. (From Narahashi, T., *Advances in Insect Physiology*, Academic Press, New York, 1971. With permission.)

firing evoked facilitatory increases in EPP amplitude which was attributed to increased ACh release (Figure 8B). Wouters and co-workers argued that the repetitive activity may be due to the ability of allethrin to prolong the transient increase in voltage-dependent sodium permeability[83,85] in the nerve terminal (Figure 9). The prolonged Na$^+$ current during excitation probably exceeds the fast rate of recovery from sodium inactivation following the first action potential and thus triggers a second action potential and so on (see Chapter 2). This theory is supported by the fact that cooling the preparation (which would increase the prolongation of the Na$^+$ current) enhances repetitive activity. Thus, allethrin appears to alter membrane conductance parameters at the nerve terminal where geometric considerations and distinctive voltage-dependent conductances may facilitate repetitive firing. This repetition is not unique to motor neurons, but has also been observed in sensory fibers.[85,109] Repetitive EPPs have also been observed by Evans[38] in frog muscle exposed to another synthetic pyrethroid compound, NRDC 119.

The effects of allethrin are quite interesting, for they alter synaptic function without a genuine ''synaptic'' effect except for repetitive activity. Neurotransmitter release, EPPs,

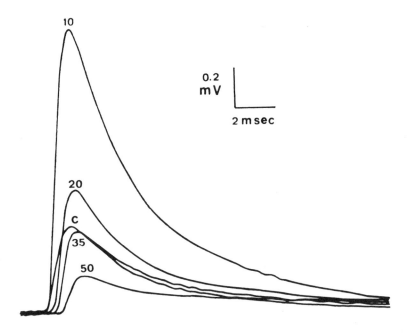

FIGURE 10. The effect of ATD on EPP amplitude in frog muscle. Computer averaged EPPs (n = 256) before (C) and at intervals after the addition of 2.5 × 10^{-5}M ATD to the bath. Note the increase in delay between the start of the sweep (stimulus artifact not shown) and the start of the EPP. Numbers indicate the time in minutes. (From Akkermans, L. M. A. et al., *Pest. Biochem. Physiol.*, 4, 313, 1974. With permission.)

and muscle responses all appear normal in the in vitro allethrin-exposed preparation, but the ability of a single impulse to generate up to 13 EPPs greatly compromises the coordinated performance of the system and may account for the in vivo neurotoxic symptoms of hyperexcitation and convulsions which may eventually lead to exhaustion, paralysis, and death.

B. Halogenated Hydrocarbons

Dieldrin (HEOD 85% w/w; 1,2,3,4,10,10-hexchloro-6,7-epoxy 1,4,4a5,6,7,8,8a-octahydro-1,4,5,8-endo-exo-dimethanonaphthalene) is a chlorinated hydrocarbon insecticide that has been shown to interfere with synaptic transmission in the CNS of the cockroach.[112] Studies on frog neuromuscular junction by Akkermanns and colleagues[3,4] indicate that dieldrin is most likely converted to an active metabolite, aldrin-transdiol (ATD; 6,7-trans-dihydroxy-dihydro-aldrin) to induce synaptic toxicity. When added to the Ringer's solution bathing the frog sartorius or EDL, ATD (2.5 × 10^{-5} M) caused a marked increase in MEPP frequency and a rapid decline in MEPP amplitude. These effects could be reversed by washing the preparation with normal medium at lower ATD doses, but were not reversible at higher concentrations of ATD (2.5 × 10^{-5} M) during low-frequency nerve stimulation (0.5 to 2 Hz). Ultimately, ATD completely blocked neuromuscular transmission. Calculations of quantal content (m) indicated increased ACh release during the transient increase in EPP amplitude, then a decrease in m in parallel to the gradual decline in amplitude (Figure 10). Iontophoretic ejection of ACh onto the end-plate recording site demonstrated that ATD, in addition to its prejunctional effects, suppressed the sensitivity of the postjunctional membrane to ACh (Figure 11).

Further studies on the active metabolite aldrin-transdiol in the frog sartorius preparation explored neuromuscular facilitation and depression by intracellular recording methods.[4] The introduction of ATD (2.5 × 10^{-5} M) in vitro enhanced facilitation transiently (7 to 10 min) corresponding to the increase in EPP amplitude previously observed (Figure 12). It is

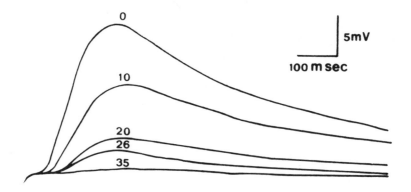

FIGURE 11. Depolarization of the end-plate membrane by ionophoretic application of ACh before (0) and at intervals (in minutes) after the application of $2.5 \times 10^{-5}M$ ATD. (From Akkermans, L. M. A. et al., *Pest. Biochem. Physiol.*, 4, 313, 1974. With permission.)

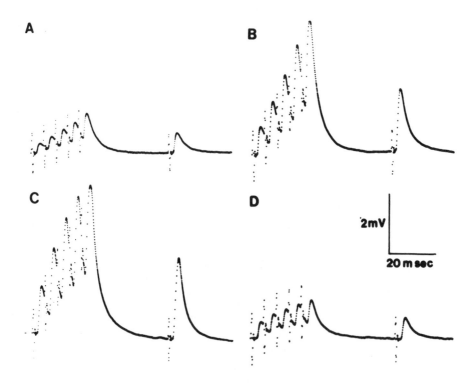

FIGURE 12. The effect of ATD on neuromuscular facilitation. EPPs were averaged by computer (n = 64) before (A) and at 7.5 (B), 10 (C) and 20 min (D) after addition of $2.5 \times 10^{-5}M$ ATD to the bath. Note the large and transient increase in EPP amplitude after ATD. (From Akkermans, L. M. A. et al., *Eur. J. Pharmacol.*, 31, 166, 1975. With permission).

noteworthy that this was observed in "blocked" preparations whose ACh release was impaired by raising Mg^{2+} and lowering Ca^{2+} concentrations in the medium. The increase in EPP amplitude was not as high when *d*-tubocurarine was used as the blocking agent. Facilitation was evoked by short trains of tetanic stimulation (five pulses at 200 Hz followed by a single stimulus at 40 msec after the train for comparison (see Figure 12); 20 min after the addition of ATD (2.5×10^{-5} *M*), EPP amplitude and the facilitatory response had declined. Since facilitation of the EPP is presumed to be due to increased transmitter release (see Chapter 3), these results support earlier conclusions that quantal ACh release is depressed

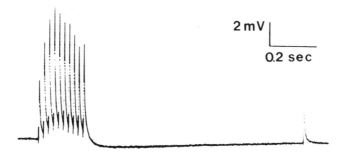

FIGURE 13. The effect of ATD on neuromuscular depression in a curarized (2×10^{-6} g/mℓ) junction. The motor nerve was stimulated with a
conditioning train of 10 pulses followed by a single test pulse (far right).
The test response in control (shown) is depressed in relation to the initial
EPP (ac coupled recording). ATD ($3 \times 10^{-5}M$) significantly enhanced
the degree of depression of the test response (not shown) from $44 \pm 5\%$
in control of $57 \pm 3\%$ depression in the presence of ATD for 12 min.
(From Akkermans, L. M. A., et al., *Eur. J. Pharmacol.*, 31, 166, 1975.
With permission).

by ATD. Moreover, the decline in facilitation after prolonged ATD treatment appeared to
be the result of an effect on neuromuscular depression.

Depression of the EPP by ATD was tested in the presence of *d*-tubocurarine (2×10^{-6}
g/mℓ) to block twitch (Figure 13). A conditioning train of ten pulses at 50 Hz was applied
to the sciatic nerve followed by a single test pulse 0.9 sec after the end of the train for
comparison. ATD enhanced the degree of depression and therefore supported the theory that
this active metabolite of dieldrin decreases evoked neurotransmitter release. The authors
speculated that initially ATD transiently increases Ca^{2+} entry during each nerve impulse;
then, after more prolonged exposure, the neurotoxicant impairs mobilization of transmitter,
thereby lowering the ACh available per impulse. Exactly how ATD interferes with maintaining a readily available pool of ACh could not be determined. Moreover, neither the
mechanism nor the extent to which ATD reduces the postjunctional effects of released ACh
were determined. Nonetheless, these studies provide experimental evidence to account for
the dieldrin-induced skeletal muscle fatigue of chronically treated rats.[56]

C. Lindane

Lindane (γ-hexachlorocyclohexane) is a chlorinated hydrocarbon insecticide that induces
in vitro acceleration of spontaneous release of ACh at the frog neuromuscular junction.[88]
Publicover and Duncan[89] showed that MEPP frequency was markedly and progressively
increased by the presence of lindane (5×10^{-5} M). MEPP amplitude gradually decreased
at a higher concentration of lindane (10^{-4} M), decreasing to 20% of control after 20 min
of exposure. These investigators suspected that the rise in MEPP frequency was due to an
increase in intraterminal $[Ca^{2+}]_i$ through increased Ca^{2+} permeability of the presynaptic
plasma membrane since the rise in MEPP frequency was reduced by lowering $[Ca^{2+}]_o$ (Figure
14). The argument was also made that like the metabolite of dieldrin, ATD, lindane increased
MEPP frequency by interfering with mitochondrial uptake of Ca^{2+} or promoting release of
Ca^{2+} from mitochondria or other organelles. Inhibition of calcium influx by lindane at
desensitized mouse neuromuscular junction lends support to this argument.[69a] The apparent
lindane-induced rise in $[Ca^{2+}]_i$ was shown in another report to be accompanied by myofi-
lament degradation and mitochondrial swelling.[88] This seems to be a recurring theme in all
studies where a neurotoxicant can be shown to augment MEPP frequency. It is reasonable
to ask whether this is a state-of-the-knowledge postulate for lack of a better understanding

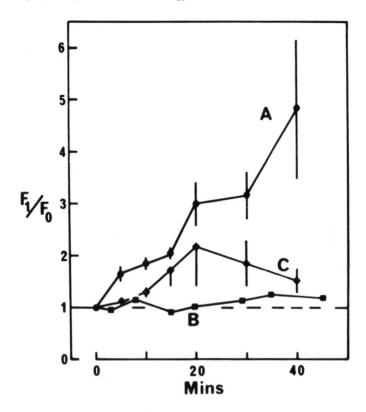

FIGURE 14.   Effect of lindane on mepp frequency at the frog neuromuscular junction at 22.5°C. $[Ca^{++}]_o = 1.8$ mM. A: $5 \times 10^{-5}M$ lindane; mean of 5 experiments; mean F_o before application of lindane equaled 82.1 MEPP/min. Calculated regression, y = 0.0876x + 1.004. B: $5 \times 10^{-6}M$ lindane (n = 1). C: $5 \times 10^{-5}M$ lindane in reduced $[Ca^{++}]_o$ of 0.5 µM (n = 5). Mean F_o equaled 28.9 MEPPs/min. Calculated regression, y = 0.0178x + 1.211. Mepp frequency (F_1) as a ratio of the control frequency (F_o) is presented on the ordinate; time after the application of lindane is presented on the abscissa. Vertical bars indicate ± SEM. (From Publicover, S. J. and Duncan, C. J., *Eur. J. Parmacol.*, 54PB, 119, 1979. With permission).

of neurobiology or whether Ca^{2+} truly plays a central role in the neurotoxic expression of diverse compounds. A comparative study of the central role of Ca^{2+} in synaptic toxicity would be a worthy subject of future investigations. Equally important would be further fundamental research on the purpose of MEPPs since the physiological significance of increased spontaneous release in vivo is unknown.

D. DDT

The chlorinated hydrocarbon insecticide, DDT, despite its notoriety, has been the subject of only a few published electrophysiological studies on synaptic toxicology. Unlike lindane, whose action is on the presynaptic terminal, DDT mainly affects axonal membranes.[82-84,97] Changes in ionic conductances (Na^+ increases and K^+ decreases) augment and prolong the depolarizing (negative) after-potential, and provoke repetitive discharges in the nerve.[83] In the first study dealing specifically with the detailed mechanism of DDT analogs on synaptic transmission, Farley and co-workers[39] studied the effects of the biodegradable analog, EDO [2,2] bis (*p*-ethoxyphenyl)-3,3-dimethyloxetane) on neuromuscular transmission in crayfish. Intracellular recordings from the claw opener muscle revealed an increase in MEPP frequency with concentrations of EDO greater than 10^{-6} M. Large, summated, repetitive EPPs were

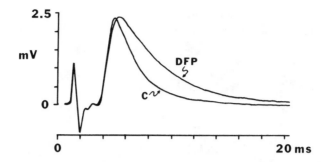

FIGURE 15. The effect of diisopropylfluorophosphate (DFP: $4 \times 10^{-5}M$) on EPPs recorded in the same cell in rat hemidiaphragm. Control tracing (C) is the average of 21 events evoked by stimulation of the phrenic nerve at 1 Hz in 1 mM Ca^{++} and 7 mM Mg^{++}. DFP caused a prolongation of the decay phase which persisted after washout of excess, unbound DFP. EPP amplitudes were not significantly affected. (From Bierkamper, G. G., *Eur. J. Pharmacol.*, 73, 343, 1981. With permission.)

observed in the presence of EDO and appeared to be due solely to repetitive firing in the nerve. In other words, the repetitive firing gave rise to greatly facilitated, prolonged EPPs, without an apparent effect on RMP, presynaptic facilitation,[4] or on postjunctional sensitivity (as shown by potentials evoked by glutamate iontophoretic application). The multiple firing induced by a single stimulus was attributed to the prolonged depolarizing afterpotential induced by EDO[83] in a manner similar to that described above for allethrin (Figure 9).[119] Tetrodotoxin blocked multiple spiking in the nerve, but failed to prevent the increase in MEPP frequency. However, increased MEPP frequency was reduced to control levels in calcium-free medium. The authors suggest that EDO has an additional effect to inducing multiple firing in the nerve to cause the increase in MEPP frequency. Since DDT is known to inhibit ATPases and also increase MEPP frequency, it was reasoned that inhibition of Na$^+$-K$^+$ ATPase might be involved in the EDO action. Unfortunately, this was not supported experimentally when 100 μM EDO was shown to have no measureable effect on Na$^+$-K$^+$ ATPase. It is clear from this study that the DDT analog, EDO, has an effect on glutaminergic transmission in the crayfish. However, it is uncertain how important these observations are to synaptic function in mammals where chronic exposure to DDT causes little apparent toxicity.[79]

E. Anticholinesterase Agents

The anticholinesterase properties of a number of compounds[69b] have made them useful for therapeutic, biocidal, and insecticidal purposes. Their primary mode of action is to inhibit acetylcholinesterase (AchE) thereby blocking the hydrolysis of ACh at the synaptic cleft. Failure to eliminate released ACh from the synaptic cleft leads to disintegration of cholinergic transmission and may be fatal to mammals and insects alike. The acute and chronic toxicity of anticholinesterase agents on neurotransmission have been widely studied due, in part, to their threat as chemical warfare agents as well as their extensive insecticidal use in agriculture. As a consequence, a large body of literature exists on the electrophysiological effects of the various reversible and irreversible cholinesterase inhibitors and has been extensively reviewed.[46]

Anticholinesterase agents alter synaptic transmission in several ways depending on the agent and the dose and length of exposure in vitro or in vivo. The predominant direct action of the anti-AChE compounds is undoubtedly postsynaptic. Inhibition of AChE causes a prolongation of the decay phase of the EPP[18,35,36,54] and end-plate currents (Figures 15 and 16).[59,60,63,64] This effect has been attributed to the persistence of unhydrolyzed ACh in the synaptic cleft and is supported by noise analysis studies in frog muscle.[54,60] Kuba and co-

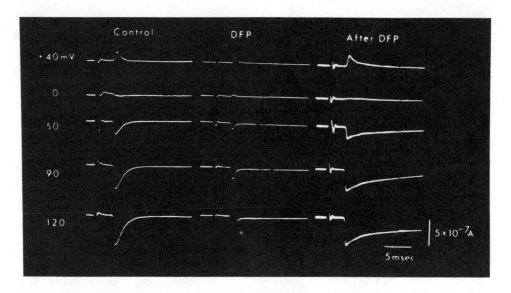

FIGURE 16.   Effects of DFP on end-plate currents recorded at different membrane potentials in the frog sartorius preparation. DFP was applied at a concentration of $1.1 \times 10^{-3}M$ for 30 min; then washed out for 30 min. Note the reversal level and the falling phase of the EPCs under different conditions. (From Kuba, K. et al., *J. Pharmacol. Exp. Therr.*, 189, 499, 1974. With permission.)

workers[64] argue that the prolongation of the decay phase may be due to the direct action of certain irreversible AChE agents, at least at high concentrations, on the ACh receptor/channel complex resulting in prolonged open channel conductances (see Review by Spivak and Albuquerque[100a]) Most AChE agents also induce a dose-dependent increase in the EPP amplitude;[18,25,35,66] however, at higher concentrations or longer exposure the EPP and EPC (end-plate current) amplitudes may be reduced.[41,63,64,106] MEPP frequency and amplitude are generally reported to be increased acutely by in vitro or in vivo anti-AChE compounds (Figure 17).[18,25,46,66,106] These acute alterations on synaptic transmission result in a well-documented and therapeutically managable clinical toxicology toxicity.[33a]

Prolonged exposure to anticholinesterases in vivo presents a different toxicological picture. This is not in reference to the delayed axonopathies of the organophosphorus compounds.[48,49] whose electrophysiological correlates at the synapse have been virtually neglected, but to (1) structural alterations in the end-plate, (2) neurally mediated myopathies, and (3) changes in cholinergic receptor density. These toxicological manifestations may have significant effects on the performance of mammalian motor systems[95,113,114] and CNS.[80]

Chang and co-workers[27] treated rats twice a day for 7 days with the reversible AChE inhibitor, neostigmine methylsulfate (0.1 mg; s.c.), then examined ACh content and release from the diaphragm. Although total ACh content was unchanged, stimulated ACh release and the total number of ACh receptors at the end-plate were reduced by approximately 50%. The authors conclude that these changes are due to the chronic accumulation of ACh at the neuromuscular junction rather than a direct effect of neostigmine. These observations were extended by a similar study employing electrophysiological methods in rat EDL muscle.[106] The same dosage regimen of neostigmine for only 3 days caused decreases in indirectly and directly elicited muscle contraction, MEPP frequency and amplitude, EPP amplitude and quantal content, and junctional ACh sensitivity. The decreased rate of transmitter release returned to nearly normal by 22 to 25 days of continued neostigmine treatment. The alterations in postsynaptic membrane persisted for over 100 days. Morphological changes were correlated with the physiological alterations. The conclusions of this study are in agreement with Laskowski et al.[66] and Chang et al.,[27] i.e., the synaptic toxicity requires functional

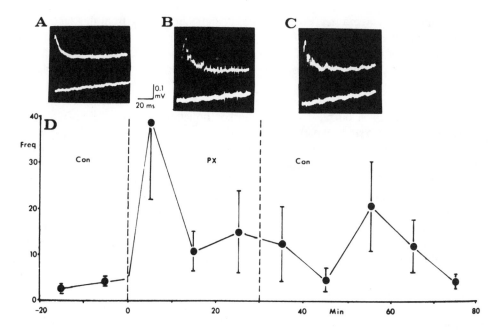

FIGURE 17.   The effect of paraoxon on MEPP frequency and antidromic activity in rat diaphragm. Dashed vertical lines enclose the 30-min period during which the preparation was perfused with $6 \times 10^{-8}M$ paraoxon (PX). A, B, and C represent evoked (upper trace) and spontaneous (lower traces) antidromic activity. A was recorded from the phrenic nerve of an untreated diaphragm. B was recorded after the application of paraoxon for 10 min. C was recorded 20 min after washout of paraoxon. D represents the mean MEPP frequency (N = 3 diaphragms) plotted as a means of 10-min intervals before, during and after perfusion of paraoxon. Time calibrations: 10 msec in B (upper trace); all others are 20 msec. (From Laskowski, M. B. and Dettbarn, W.-D., *J. Parmacol. Exp. Ther.*, 194, 351, 1975. With permission.)

motor nerves and is unlikely to result from a direct effect of neostigmine. The thorough and scholarly nature of the report by Tiedt and co-workers,[106] although not designed to address directly an environmental chemical, is a worthy model for other electrophysiological studies on synaptic toxicology and is presented here in the anticipation that future electrophysiologically oriented studies will comply to a similar rigorous and informative design.

Similar toxicological results have been reported for organophosphate anticholinesterases of environmental interest.[65-68,94,114] Laskowski and Dettbarn[66] studied the effects of paraoxon, the active metabolite of parathion, in isolated hemidiaphragm muscles removed from rats previously injected. Neuromuscular cholinesterase activity was reduced to 36% of control in hemidiaphragms dissected from rats 30 min after i.p. injection with paraoxon (0.5 mg/ kg). Intracellular recordings from these preparations demonstrated a marked increase in MEPP frequency (109/sec vs. 2.9/sec control) at the 30-min postinjection time point. This increase was reduced in Ca^{2+}-free medium and was antagonized by elevated Mg^{2+} concentrations. The increased MEPP frequency gradually returned to normal after 6 hr in the bath, despite persistent cholinesterase inhibition. Quantal content was significantly reduced by paraoxon pretreatment, although the amplitude of the first EPP in a train and quantum size were increased. Quantum size was estimated by dividing the variance of EPPs 21 to 40 in a train (5 Hz) by the mean EPP amplitude of the same EPP sequence. It is unfortunate that the authors neither discussed the usefulness of this parameter, nor the significance of the inverse relationship observed between quantal content and quantum size. Tetrodotoxin and pyridine-2-aldoxime methiodide (2-PAM) antagonized the effect of paraoxon on MEPP frequency. Laskowski and Dettbarn[65] also demonstrated spontaneous and evoked antidromic nerve action potentials, muscle fasciculations, and muscle fiber necrosis, and raised questions about the direct or indirect effects of paraoxon. A subsequent study from this laboratory[67] revealed, by electron microscopy, structural abnormalities in the sarcoplasm beneath the end-plate as part of the myopathy. Taken together, these studies strongly suggest that the ability of paraoxon to inhibit cholinesterase is the primary action to account for changes at the neuromuscular junction.

Another electrophysiological study by Laskowski and Dettbarn[65] concentrated on the in vitro effects of paraoxon on rat diaphragm. In conformation of their preliminary studies associated with the 1975 study,[66] paraoxon (0.6 μM) was shown to increase MEPP frequency, to prolong the MEPP decay phase, and to produce antidromic activity. Curiously, muscle membrane was more depolarized around the end-plate, an effect of paraoxon (10^{-5} M) reversible by 10 μM d-tubocurarine. High Mg^{2+} also blocked the exaggerated end-plate depolarization, presumably by lowering ACh release. The effects of paraoxon were all shown to be dose dependent, i.e., related to the degree of AChE inhibition. Reactivation of cholinesterase with 2-PAM reversed the effects of paraoxon on synaptic transmission. Paraoxon concentrations of 10^{-5} to 10^{-3} M produced irreversible muscle block. The authors conclude that both the in vivo and in vitro effects of paraoxon are due to AChE inhibition and the resultant ACh in the cleft.

AChE-induced antidromic activity (backfiring) has recently been addressed by Aizenman and co-workers[1,2] in the vascular perfused mouse phrenic nerve-hemidiaphragm (Figure 18). Backfiring was shown to require the release of ACh from nerve terminal. A direct effect of the AChE agent, neostigmine, was ruled out by blocking ACh release with botulinum and tetanus toxin; backfiring could also be elicited with vascular perfusion of ACh even in the absence of AChE inhibition. Moreover, backfiring was blocked by d-tubocurarine. The ACh-mediated backfiring was argued to be due to action of cleft ACh on prejunctional nicotinic cholinoceptors whose activation induces depolarization changes in the nerve terminal.[2] These studies support the conclusions of Laskowski and Dettbarn, that the effects of the anticholinesterase agents, including backfiring, are due to excessive, unhydrolyzed ACh residing in the cleft after nerve stimulation.

Wecker et al.[113,114] studied the effects of paraoxon in neuromuscular tissue removed from treated rats. A dose-dependent paraoxon myopathy was induced if at least 85% AChE inhibition was obtained within the 1st hr of injection (0.23 mg/kg with 2-PAM and atropine protection). Prophylactic administration of reversible AChE inhibitors (e.g., physostigmine and neostigmine) prevented muscle necrosis. Thus, the results indicated that both the degree and duration of AChE inhibition are critical to the necrotic process. In an overview of their studies, the authors[114] conclude that repeated transmitter-receptor interactions (hyperactivity) as a result of a critically severe degree of AChE inhibition causes the loss of muscle fiber integrity and induces the necrotic myopathy. These conclusions are substantially strengthened by a subsequent histological study by Salpeter and colleagues[95] in which excessive levels of the nonhydrolyzable cholinergic agonist, carbachol (10^{-4} M) in vitro, showed morphological changes similar to that with the AChE organophosphate compounds.[69] The results were interpreted to indicate that the anticholinesterase-induced muscle necrosis is most likely due to persistence of ACh at the synaptic nicotinic receptor sites which causes the accumulation of abnormally high levels of Ca^{2+} in the end-plate region. The accumulated Ca^{2+} would enter the muscle cells via the ionic conductance channels of the AChR and activate proteases which would break down certain muscle proteins. Sites like the sarcoplasmic reticulum would be damaged in attempts to lower the excessive Ca^{2+} levels.[34] This is a very interesting hypothesis that toxicological induction of synaptic hyperactivity may lead to neuroeffector cell damage and deserves further correlative examination with electrophysiological methods.

Chronic exposure to non-necrotizing concentrations of organophosphate insecticides has been shown to result in significant changes in cholinergic receptor density at the synapse.

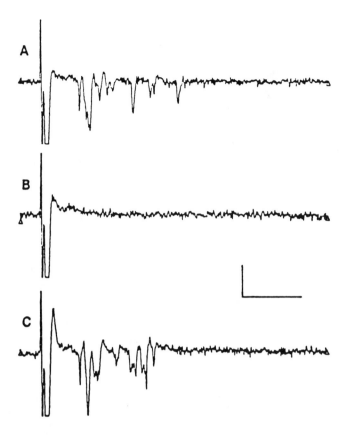

FIGURE 18. The effect of nicotinic antagonism on stimulus-induced antidromic activity (sADA) in mouse phrenic nerve-hemidiaphragm. Responses were recorded from the phrenic nerve following the delivery of a single stimulus. A: response recorded 2 min after infusion of 2 μM neostigmine via the cannulated vascular system. B: response after addition of trimethaphan camsylate (20 μM). C: response following washout of the antagonist. Vertical bar = 0.05 mV; horizontal bar represent 10 msec. (From Aizenman, E. et al., *J. Physiol.*, 372, 395, 1986. With permission.)

This has been summarily addressed in a recent chapter by Murphy et al.[80] and will not be discussed here. The point to be made, however, is that the brief in vitro administration of a neurotoxic compound may yield strikingly different results to the effects observed after subchronic in vivo exposure. The well-studied anti-AChE agents should serve as a model of caution and anticipation in neurotoxicological studies on other compounds.

OTHER NEUROTOXIC COMPOUNDS

A. Dithiobiuret

2,4-Dithiobiuret (dithioimidodicarbonic diamide; DTB, H_2N-CS - NH-CS-NH_2) is a synthesized thiourea derivative whose reducing properties have application in the chemical industry and whose use as a pesticide has been proposed by virtue of its biocidal properties. Subchronic administration of DTB produces a delayed - onset, flaccid muscular weakness.[8,14] Atchison, Peterson and co-workers have made an extensive study of the toxicokinetics and neuromuscular toxicity of DTB.[14,15,85,116] DTB treatment (1 mg/kg/day; i.p. for 6 days) of rats depressed twitch tension, caused tetanic fade, and altered post-tetanic potentiation in contractile experiments in the sciatic nerve-gastrocnemius preparation *in situ*.[9] This series

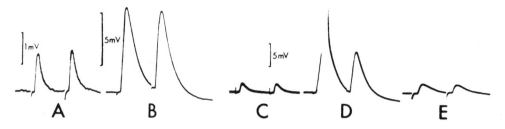

FIGURE 19. The effects of ethanol on neurotransmission at rat neuromuscular junction. EPPs recorded at 10 msec intervals in curarized junctions ($2.3 \times 10^{-6}M$ d-tubocurarine). A: in control medium. B: after 18 sec in 1.25 M ethyl alcohol. C: another control junction. D: after 4 sec in 1.25 M ethyl alcohol. E. after 3 min in control medium. The change in stimulus artifact was caused by increasing the stimulus intensity. Recordings were made at 34°C. (From Gage, P. W., *J. Pharmacol. Exp. Ther.*, 150, 236, 1965. With permission.)

of experiments suggested a defect in neuromuscular transmission of a prejunctional origin. A subsequent study of muscle contraction provided indirect evidence to support the theory that DTB has a prejunctional effect.[10] The ability of 4-aminopyridine to reverse the DTB-induced depression of contractile tension was interpreted to indicate that DTB may reduce quantal ACh release. Recent preliminary experiments by Atchison[123] reveal a slight reduction in EPP amplitude as measured in EDL muscle of DTB-treated rats (1 mg/kg/day; 6 days, i.p.). In EDL preparations from severely paralyzed subjects, subthreshold EPPs could be recorded without the need for curare or altered Ca^{2+}/Mg^{2+} to prevent twitch. These preliminary experiments strengthen the argument that DTB induces muscle weakness by altering neurotransmission. However, broadening of the MEPPs and insufficient data to calculate the statistical parameters of release make it difficult at this time to confirm a purely pre-synaptic locus of DTB neurotoxicity. Nonetheless, the sequence of studies on dithiobiuret by Atchison and colleagues provides an exemplary multidisciplinary design for investigating a compound of suspected synaptic toxicity. Moreover, the numerous *indirect* observations suggesting prejunctional toxicity emphasize the importance of applying, at some point, an electrophysiological technique as a powerful means of directly determining the action of a toxicant on the realtime, dynamic state of neurotransmission.

B. Aliphatic Alcohols

Observations on the effects of aliphatic alcohols on neuromuscular transmission offer fundamental knowledge for understanding the acute actions of other potentially neurotoxic aliphatic solvents. Gage[42] conducted the first intracellular recording experiments on isolated rat hemidiaphragm preparations to test the in vitro action of methyl, ethyl, and *N*-propyl alcohols. In curarized preparations, molar concentrations of ethanol (approximately 5% solutions) increased EPP amplitude sixfold and prolonged the time course. However, this response was transient and after approximately 1 min of 100-Hz test stimulation, nerve block occurred and EPPs failed (Figure 19). Washout of ethanol with normal medium reversed the block. MEPP amplitude and time course were also increased at higher concentrations. The effect of ethanol on the EPP was primarily presynaptic as evidenced by an increase in quantal content and a partial depletion of the immediately available store of transmitter. The prolongation of the EPP by ethanol was argued to pertain to changes in the physical properties of the muscle membrane. This is an especially cogent argument in view of the historical context of the early sixties when a paucity of experimental evidence existed on the physical properties of biomembranes and lipid bilayers.

More reasonable concentrations of ethanol (8 and 16 mM) were subsequently examined in magnesium-blocked preparations in an attempt to differentiate pre- and postsynaptic actions.[42] Again, the quantal content of EPPs was increased (2.3 control vs. 3.3 after 8 min

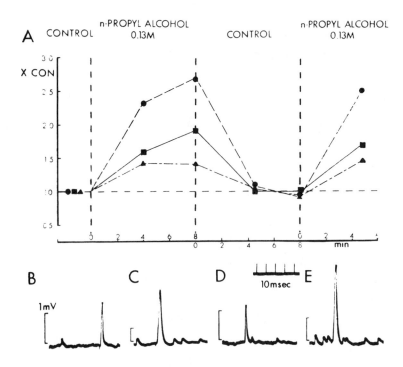

FIGURE 20.   The effect of 0.13 *M* *n*-propanol on EPP amplitude (solid circles), MEPPs (solid triangles) and the quantal content of EPPs (solid squares). A: ordinate: ratio of sizes of the initial average size in control solution before exposure to *n*-propyl alcohol. B, C, D, and E: An average EPP with MEPPs is shown in each trace. B: In control solution; C: after 8 min of *n*-propanol; D: after 8 min in control medium; E: after 5 min in *n*-propyl alcohol. Vertical calibration equals 1 mV. MgCl$_2$ was present at 14 m*M* to prevent contraction; recordings were made at 35°C. (From Gage, P. W., *J. Pharmacol. Exp. Ther.*, 150, 236, 1965. With permission.)

of ethanol), but without altering MEPP amplitude or the postsynaptic response. Concentrations of ethyl alcohol above 16 m*M* caused both pre- and postsynaptic effects. The enhancement of EPP amplitude and the increased time course were directly dose related, and were limited by eventual blocking of nerve conduction at higher concentrations of ethanol. The postsynaptic effect of ethanol resembled AChE inhibition (increased MEPP amplitude and prolongation of the decay phase of the EPPs). However, neostigmine ($3.3 \times 10^{-6}M$) did not prevent the 0.16-*M* ethanol-induced rise in MEPP amplitude (attributed by Gage to a postjunctional mechanism), and thus ruled out cholinesterase inhibition. Measurement of the input resistance of a large number of muscle fibers before and after exposure to ethanol showed a reversible mean increase from 0.56 ± 0.01 to 0.62 ± 0.01 MΩ respectively. Hence, according to the work of Katz and Thesleff,[35] the increase in input resistance could, at least partially, account for the increase in MEPP amplitude. Methyl and *n*-propyl alcohol had similar effects to ethanol on potentiating EPP and MEPP amplitudes and increasing quantal content (Figure 20).

   An additional postjunctional action was determined to affect the performance of the neuromuscular preparation. Ethanol (0.2 *M*) caused a slight, reversible decline in isometric tetanic tension in isolated toad sartorius muscle.[42] This was interpreted to mean that ethanol has a negative effect on the contractile mechanism of the muscle fiber. A more recent investigation on the in vivo effects of ethanol demonstrated a delay in nerve-to-muscle impulse transmission (increased residual latency interval) at concentrations as low as 1.0 g ethanol per kilogram i.p. The effect was attributed to combined delays in action potential propagation on both sides of the synapse.

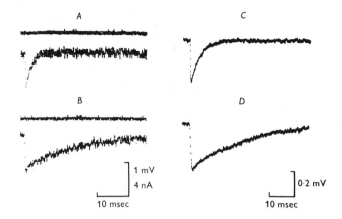

FIGURE 21.   Prolongation of MEPCs caused by ethanol. Records A
(standard solution) and B (0.5 *M* ethanol solution) were obtained in a
voltage-clamped fiber from toad neuromuscular junction. Traces C (standard solution) and D (0.5 *M* ethanol solution) were recorded extracellularly.
Calibrations for A and B = 1 mV, 4 nA vertical and 10 msec horizontal;
for C and D = 0.2 mV vertical and 10 msec horizontal. (From Gage, P.
W. et al., *J. Physiol.*, 244, 409, 1975. With permission.)

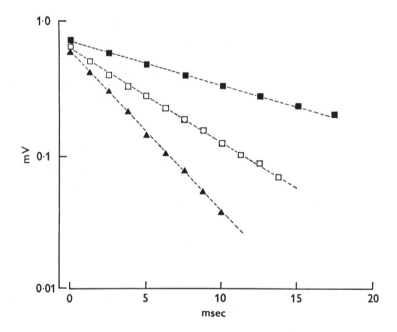

FIGURE 22.   The exponential decay of MEPCs recorded extracellularly in one fiber for
3 different concentrations of ethanol: 0.125 *M* (triangles), 0.25 *M* (open squares), and
0.5 *M* (solid squares). The ordinate is logarithmic. (From Gage, P. W. et al., *J. Physiol.*,
244, 409, 1975. With permission.)

Gage and co-workers[43] continued their electrophysiological study of the aliphatic alcohols,
ethanol to hexanol, on toad neuromuscular junction. By voltage clamp technology, they
determined that the alcohol-induced increase in MEPP amplitude and duration was due to
the prolongation of the decay phase of miniature end-plate currents (MEPCs; Figure 21) in
a dose-dependent manner (Figure 22). A linear relationship was described between the time
constant of the decay of MEPCs and the carbon chain length of the alcohol. The observed

prolongation of the MEPC is an important finding for the rate of the decay phase of the synaptic current is a crucial determinant of the "throughput" capacity of the synapse *in situ*. The results of this work, therefore, favor the theory that alcohols act by changing the dielectric constant of the postsynaptic membrane. This perturbation provides the environment for the rate-limiting events responsible for the decay of the ACh-induced conductances in the end-plate. Moreover, the rate-limiting process during the decay of the MEPCs is argued to be a first-order, voltage-sensitive chemical reaction involving dipoles occurring in the lipid environment in the postsynaptic membrane. These dipoles are thought to be associated with channel gating. According to these investigators, the shorter-chain alcohols seem to act on the polarizability of membrane in the vicinity of the channel whereas, the more hydrophobic, longer-chain alcohols probably increase the membrane fluidity near the channel. Therefore, changes in the regional dipoles or perturbation of the lipid membrane environment by the aliphatic alcohols is postulated to alter channel gating and prolong the MEPC.

The changes described by Gage and colleagues may not be directly extrapolatable to other synapses as shown by Wachtel.[111] She found a faster rate of decay of the end-plate currents (EPCs) at the crayfish neuromuscular junction in response to in vitro exposure of ethanol to octanol. The potency of each alcohol in increasing the rate of decay of the currents was demonstrated to be exponentially related to carbon chain length. Paradoxically, these experiments support Gage's hypothesis that the aliphatic alcohols cause changes in membrane polarizability and fluidity. If ACh-activated currents at the amphibian end-plate are prolonged by short-chain alcohols, which do indeed alter membrane polarizability, then they should have the opposite effects in toads and in crayfish due to the opposite orientation of the dipoles in the two preparations. Wachtel's experiments on glutamate-induced EPCs support this hypothesis. Consequently, ethanol through octanol shorten the decay phase of the EPCs at the crayfish neuromuscular junction by interactions with the lipid phase of the membrane (fluidity). A comparison of the earlier experiments of Gage[42,43] on the amphibian with the recent experiments of Wachtel on the crayfish emphasizes the potential toxicological differences to be found between species and between neuronal systems. Moreover, it demonstrates the ability to predict toxicological perturbations from system to system when basic information is available from previous studies of mindful design.

These experiments also provide useful information to investigators who find it necessary to dissolve hydrophobic test compounds in ethanolic solutions inasmuch as the vehicle is likely to have an independent or additive effect.

C. 2,5 Hexanedione

The neurotoxic solvents, methyl-*n*-butyl ketone and *n*-hexane, have been shown to produce a distal axonopathy through a common metabolite, 2,5-hexanedione.[32,99] In one of the rare electrophysiological studies in which a neurotoxicant was administered in vivo, Cangiano and co-workers examined the early stages of synaptic toxicity induced by subchronic 2,5-hexanedione exposure. Adult male rats were injected with 2,5-hexanedione exposure. Adult male rats were injected with 2,5-hexanedione (450 mg/kg/day or less) for up to 34 days. Clinical signs of neuropathy (e.g., muscle weakness and ataxia) were evident between 13 and 18 days of treatment. The effect of this treatment on neuromuscular transmission was investigated using conventional intracellular recording methods in the isolated soleus and EDL muscles. RMP, MEPPs, and EPPs were recorded in the presence of *d*-tubocurarine (0.5×10^{-6} g/mℓ). These experiments had the added complication that EPP could not be recorded from chemically denervated muscle. Consequently, fibers without EPPs were designated as *denervated* (Table 1). Surprisingly, no decrease in RMP was reported in the "denervated" myofibers[101] until examination of the 34-day exposure group. This group exhibited a 10% decrease in the RMP of EDL. Morphological changes were observed at

Table 1
ELECTROPHYSIOLOGICAL EXAMINATION (AT NEUROMUSCULAR JUNCTIONS) OF MUSCLE FIBERS OF RATS TREATED FOR 2 WEEKS WITH 2,5-HEXANEDIONE

	EDL		Soleus	
	Normal	Treated	Normal	Treated
Percent of fibers without transmitted A.P.[a] and EPP	0%	22%	0%	6%
Mean quantal content ($\pm$ SE) of the EPP[b]	385 $\pm$ 74	146 $\pm$ 16*	254 $\pm$ 51	217 $\pm$ 33
Frequency (sec^{-1} $\pm$ SE) MEPPs[c]	1.80 $\pm$ 0.12	2.66 $\pm$ 0.21*	1.53 $\pm$ 0.11	2.32 $\pm$ 0.28*
Amplitude (μV $\pm$ SE)	382 $\pm$ 26	512 $\pm$ 29*	450 $\pm$ 26	586 $\pm$ 48**
RMP[d] (mv $\pm$ SE)	76.4 $\pm$ 0.8	74.3 $\pm$ 0.5	72.0 $\pm$ 0.7	73.6 $\pm$ 0.6

Note: Each value refers to 20 to 30 fibers from 3 to 6 muscles. The statistical significance between the difference of the mean values of treated vs. normal muscles was tested with Student's *t*-test; * = p < 0.001, ** = p < 0.02.

[a]   A.P.: action potential.
[b]   EPP: end-plate potential.
[c]   MEPP: miniature end-plate potential.
[d]   RMP: resting membrane potential.

the neuromuscular junction (soleus) prior to evidence of the stereotypic axonal lesions in the peripheral nerves (giant axonopathy).

Fourteen days of 2,5-hexadione treatment increased MEPP frequency and amplitude in both EDL and soleus;[26] 22% of the myofibers in EDL failed to produce an EPP on nerve stimulation; soleus had 6% not responding. In addition, mean quantal content was significantly reduced in EDL, but not soleus. Curiously, the denervated fibers responded to directly elicited action potentials (double microelectrode techniques) with only a slight reduction in response in the presence of TTX (10^{-6}) which normally abolished the response of healthy fibers.[91] The authors concluded that progressive functional impairment of the neuromuscular junction precedes the typical axonal lesions induced by 2,5-hexanedione. The transient increase in MEPP frequency, followed by disappearance, has been described after surgical denervation.[118] The decrease in quantal content implies an impairment of phasic ACh release, perhaps due to early denervation changes such as, in theory, partial depolarization of the nerve terminal. This has also been a common supposition in other studies where an impairment in neuronal metabolism was suspected of causing depolarization changes (hypoxia,[47] dicoumarol,[7] dinitrophenol,[44,62] and triethyltin[75]). The differential effects of 2,5-hexanedione on fast (EDL) and slow (soleus) muscle fibers strengthen the argument of a bioenergetic defect.[21,92] Based on the cautiously preliminary results (but plausible hypothesis) of Sabri et al.,[93] Cangiano and colleagues suggested that inhibition of glycolytic enzymes may compromise the functional capacity of the motor neurons, leading to inhibition of the Na$^+$-K$^+$-ATPase (sodium pump) and membrane depolarization. The consequent depolarization and/or additional deficiencies in bioenergetic capacity within the nerve terminal would be expected to reduce evoked neurotransmitter release.[20] Bierkamper and Bassett[21] have reported a unique model system for the investigation of bioenergetic pathways in the dynamically functioning hemidiaphragm preparation which would be of value in continued studies on this hypothesis. Despite the logical, moderately supported case for bioenergetic impairment, other factors such as membrane composition changes[81] should not be neglected in future electrophysiological experiments.

V. CONCLUSIONS

Several observations are striking in reviewing the literature on the synaptic toxicology of environmental agents as studied by electrophysiological methods: (1) there are relatively few studies published, (2) the published studies predominantly examined only the in vitro effects of the agent, (3) the isolated biological preparations used in most studies are derived from the peripheral nerve and skeletal muscles of rodents or amphibians, (4) most investigations use intracellular recording of EPPs as the primary technique, (5) there are few studies which actually exploit the power of electrophysiological methods or use multidisciplinary techniques in determining mechanism of action, (6) there are a relatively few number of compounds that have been studied thoroughly enough to understand their acute (in vitro and in vivo) and chronic (in vivo) toxicity, (7) few studies are reported using electrophysiological techniques to study the reversibility of toxic insult by removal of the agent or by therapeutic measures, (8) most of the compounds studied appear to have predominantly presynaptic actions (this is probably due, in part to methodological selection and bias), and (9) interference with Ca^{2+} or calcium mismanagement within the nerve terminal are the common arguments for why environmental agents alter neurotransmitter release.

The most disappointing factor of the majority of the reviewed studies is that the investigators rarely correlated their in vitro data with the in vivo consequences of toxicity. Furthermore, the assumption is repeatedly made that the peripheral neurons or neuromuscular junctions represent good models of extrapolation for the toxicity of CNS, yet few reports experimentally address this issue. One also finds that correlation with other studies, e.g., biochemical and histological, is often neglected, thus limiting the depth of interpretation of a given paper.

The electrophysiological dissection of synaptic toxicity described in this review reveals several general pre- and postsynaptic targets whose identification provides a clearer understanding of the mechanism of neurotoxicity of selected environmental agents. These mechanisms include

1. Competition for the voltage-dependent Ca^{2+} sites or channels on the nerve terminal which are associated with neurotransmitter release (e.g., Pb^{2+}, mercury, Cd^{2+}, and other polyvalent cations). Antagonism of this site is most often reflected in a reduction of EPP amplitude and a concomitant decrease in the statistical parameters of release, *m* and *n*. Moreover, evidence exists that these cations may enter the cell through voltage-dependent channels including those for Na^+, K^+, and Ca^{2+} and affect intracellular processes.
2. Interference with intraterminal Ca^{2+} sequestration and/or release (buffering processes) associated with intracellular organelles such as mitochondria (e.g., lead, mercury, TET, and lindane). The mechanisms may involve a block in transport of cations across the mitochondrial membrane or direct damage to mitochondrial integrity. Intraterminal Ca^{2+} mismanagment appears to be reflected in changes in spontaneous transmitter release, particularly in the absence of external Ca^{2+}. Postulated increases in intraterminal Ca^{2+} by various agents cause elevations in MEPP frequency, sometimes to dramatic rates and for long durations in vitro. On the other hand, agents which transiently increase MEPP frequency (Hg) may also block spontaneous release. The ability to stimulate Hg-blocked spontaneous release with La^{3+}[13] suggests a more complicated mechanism and presents the need for more detailed toxicological studies on the synaptic effects of intraterminal Ca^{2+} mismangment, especially during subchronic in vivo exposure paradigms.

3.   Interference with the neurotransmitter mobilization and release mechanism. Dieldrin and Hg were shown to alter the ability of the nerve terminals to mobilize neurotransmitter stores and/or maintain a readily releasable pool. The effect of mercury can be argued to involve sulfhydryl reactions along the mobilization and release pathway. The overall effect of interference at this site is to depress quantal release and ultimately to block neurotransmission.

4.   Direct actions on membrane structure, fluidity, and/or excitability. A number of environmental agents (e.g., aliphatic alcohols, pyrethroids, organotin compounds, and halogenated hydrocarbons) appear to alter membrane premeability in a manner detrimental to neuronal firing. Allethrin has been shown to cause repetitive, facilitated EPPs after one stimulus. This phenomenon is postulated to involve a prolongation of the Na^+ currents peculiar to the nerve terminal region such that the repetitive activity remains a local event. Changes in ionic conductances have also been described for aliphatic alcohols, DDT and its analogs, and organotin compounds. The alcohols appear to alter membrane fluidity by inserting into the lipid matrix. DDT and its analogs induce repetitive firing by altering ionic conductance and prolonging the negative afterpotential. Triethyltin acts as an anionic carrier in membranes and alters the permeability of both the plasma and mitochondrial membranes. These reversible physicochemical alterations in membrane function may not be long tolerated by the cell and have been shown to lead to failure of neurotransmission and ultrastructural changes in the neuron.

5.   Compromises in the bioenergetic pathways of the neuron. Neurotransmission is an energy-intensive process as reflected by the high density of mitochondria in the vicinity of the synapse. TET and Hg have been shown to inhibit mitochondrial oxidative phosphorylation; 2,5 hexanedione inhibits glycolytic enzymes in the neuron. A compromise in the bioenergetic capacity of the cell has been invoked to explain decreases in mepp and Epp amplitudes and quantal content as a result of poisoning with these agents. Often the deficiencies in bioenergetic capacity become most apparent in vitro when the preparation is driven by a demanding physiological stimulation rate. These deficiencies are apparent in the intact animal as manifested by muscular weakness, ataxia, and lethargy.

6.   Interactions with the postjunctional receptor and/or its membrane environment. The anticholinesterase agents and mercury have been shown to interact with the postjunctional receptor complexes as reflected in changes in postjunctional sensitivity to the transmitter and distortion of the postsynaptic potential. Hg^{2+} is postulated to bind to the −SH groups of the receptor complex; DFP is argued to interfere with the receptor associated ion channel.

7.   Inhibition of AChE at the neuromuscular junction. The anti-AChE agents distort synaptic trasmission by preventing the normal post-stimulus hydrolysis of ACh. This is reflected in increased MEPP and EPP amplitudes and a prolongation of the decay phase of both potentials. Higher concentrations of these agents may provoke postjunctional receptor desensitization and may block neuromuscular transmission either through a depolarization block or by virtue of a direct effect on the postjunctional receptor complexes.

8.   Induction of transmitter-induced changes in the postjunctional cell by anticholinesterase-induced hyperactivity. Excessive residual transmitter at the neuromuscular junction appears to have a profound effect on the postjunctional cell in vitro and in vivo. High concentrations of ACh and its nonhydrolyzable analogs have been shown to induce a necrotic myopathy in the endplate regions of skeletal muscles. This is an unusual neurotoxicity induced by overactivity of the neurotransmitter, rather than the more commonly described presynaptic alterations in neurotransmitter release.

The ability of electrophysiological methods (primarily intracellular recording) to elucidate these different target sites of toxicity at the synapse illustrates the invaluable nature of these techniques. The limited number of studies using these techniques to examine the synaptic toxicology of environmentsl agents attests to their underutilization. Further, the scarcity of electrophysiological investigations into the synaptic effects of *chronic* exposure of environmental chemicals importunes an escalation of investigational effort as a means of obtaining a full description of their peripheral and central neurotoxicity. Through the knowledge gained from this work, one would anticipate the development of new therapeutic measures, an improvement in our ability to predict neurotoxicology, and an advancement of our understanding of neuropathological processes.

ACKNOWLEDGEMENTS

The helpful suggestions of Drs. William Atchinson and Elias Aizenman are gratefully acknowledged. This review and the author's research in neuromuscular toxicology have been supported in part by NIEHS grants ES03331 and ESO4248.

REFERENCES

1. **Aizenman, E. Stanley, E. F., and Bierkamper, G. G.,** Axonally transported alpha-bungarotoxin binding sites as a putative mechanism for motor nerve backfiring, *Proc. West. Pharmacol. Soc.,* 28, 201, 1985.
2. **Aizenman, E., Bierkamper, G. G., and Stanley, E. F.,** Effect of botulinum toxin on stimulus-induced antidromic activity by nesostimgine in mouse phrenic nerve-hemidiaphragm, *J. Physiol.,* 372, 395, 1986.
3. **Akkermans, L. M. A., van den Bercken, J., van der Zalm, J. M., and van Straaten, H. W. M.,** Effects of dieldrin (HEOD) and some of its metabolites on synaptic transmission in the frog motor endplate, *Pest. Biochem. Physiol.,* 4, 313, 1974.
4. **Akkermans, L. M.A., van den Bercken, J., and van der Zalm, J. M.,** Effects of aldrin-transdiol on neuromuscular facilitation and depression, *Eur. J. Pharmacol.,* 31, 166, 1975.
5. **Aldridge, W. N. and Street, B. W.,** Oxidative phosphorylation: the relation between specific binding of trimethyltin and triethyltin to mitochondria and their effect on various mitochondrial functions, *Biochem. J.,* 124, 221, 1971.
5a. **Alkadhi, K. A. and Taha, M, N.,** Antagonism by calcium of the inhibitory effect of methylmercury on sympathetic ganglia, *Arch. Toxicol.,* 51, 175, 1982.
6. **Allen, J. E., Gage, P. W., Leaver, D. D., and Leow, A. C. T.,** Triethyltin depresses evoked transmitter release at the mouse neuromuscular junction, *Chem. Biol. Interact.,* 31, 227, 1980.
7. **Alnaes, E. and Rahamimoff, R.,** On the role of mitochondria in transmitter release from motor nerve terminals, *J. Physiol.,* 248, 285, 1975.
8. **Astwood, E. B., Hughes, A. M., Lubin, M., Vanderlaan, W. P., and Adams, R. D.,** Reversible paralysis of motor function in rats from the chronic administration of dithiobiuret, *Science,* 102, 196, 1945.
9. **Atchison, W. D., Lalley, P. M., Cassens, R. G., and Peterson, R. E.,** Depression of neuromuscular function in the rat by chronic 2,4-dithiobiuret treatment, *Neurotoxicology,* 2, 329, 1981.
10. **Atchison, W. D., Mellon, W. S., Lalley, P. M., and Peterson, R. E.,** Dithiobiuret-induced muscle weakness in rats: evidence for a prejunctional effect, *Neurotoxicology,* 3, 44, 1982.
11. **Atchison, W. D. and Narahashi, T.,** Methylmercury-induced depression of neuromuscular transmission in the rat, *Neurotoxicology,* 3, 37, 1982.
12. **Atchison, W. D. and Narahashi, T.,** Mechanisms of action of lead on neuromuscular junctions, *Neurotoxicology,* 5, 267, 1984.
13. **Atchison, W. D., Clark, A. W., and Narahashi, T.,** Presynaptic effects of methylmercury at the mammalian neuromuscular junction, *Cellular and Molecular Neurotoxicology,* Narahashi, T., Ed., Raven Press, New York, 1984, 23.
14. **Atchison, W. D. and Peterson, R. E.,** Potential neuromuscular toxicity of 2,4-dithiobiuret in the rat, *Toxicol. Appl. Pharmacol.,* 57, 63, 1981.
15. **Atchison, W. D., Yang, K. H., and Peterson, R. E.,** Dithiobiuret toxicity in the rat: evidence for latency and cumulative dose thresholds, *Toxicol. Appl. Pharmacol.,* 61, 166, 1981.

16. **Audesirk, G. and Audesirk, T.,** Effects of chronic low level lead exposure on the physiology of individually identifiable neurons, *Neurotoxicology,* 4, 13, 1983.

17. **Barnes, J. M. and Stoner, H. B.,** The toxicology of tin compounds, *Pharmacol. Rev.,* 11, 211, 1959.

17a. **Barrett, J., Botz, D., and Change, D. B.,** Block of neuromuscular transmission of methylmercury, in *Behavior Toxicology: Early Detection of Occupational Hazards,* Xintaras, C., Johnson, B. L., and de Groot, I., Eds., U.S. Department of Health, Education and Welfare, 1974, 277.

18. **Bierkamper, G. G.,** Electrophysiological effects of diisopropylfluorophosphate on neuromuscular transmission, *Eur. J. Pharmacol.,* 73, 343, 1981.

19. **Bierkamper, G. G. and Aizenman, E.,** Cholinergic agonist and antagonist interactions on the putative nicotinic cholinoceptor of motor neurons, *Proc. West. Pharmacol. Soc.,* 27, 353, 1984.

20. **Bierkamper, G. G., Aizenman, E., and Millington, W. R.,** Neuromuscular function and organotin compounds, *Neurotoxicology,* 5, 245, 1984.

21. **Bierkamper, G. G. and Bassett, D. J. P.,** Is triethyltin-induced muscular dysfunction a result of mitochondrial compromise?, in *Cellular and Molecular Neurotoxicology,* Narahashi, T., Ed., Raven Press, New York, 1984, 109.

22. **Bierkamper, G. G. and Valdes, J. J.,** Triethyltin intoxication alters acetylcholine release from rat phrenic nerve-hemidiaphragm, *Neurobehav. Toxicol. Teratol.,* 4, 251, 1982.

23. **Binah, O., Meiri, U., and Rahamimoff, H.,** The effects of mercuric chloide and mersalylon mechanisms regulating intracellular calcium and transmitter release, *Eur. J. Pharmacol.,* 51, 453, 1978.

24. **Blioch, Z. L., Glagoleva, I. M., Liberman, E. A., and Nenashev, V. A.,** A study of the mechanism of quantal transmitter release at a chemical synapse, *J. Physiol. (London),* 199, 11, 1968.

25. **Bois, R. T., Hummel, R. G., Dettbarn, W.-D., and Laskowski, M. B.,** Presynaptic and postsnyaptic neuromuscular effects of a specific inhibitor of acetylcholinesterase, *J. Pharmacol. Exp. Ther.,* 215, 53, 1980.

26. **Cangiano, A., Lutzemberger, L., Rizzuto, N., Simonati, A., Rossi, A., and Toschi, G.,** Neurotoxic effects of 2,5-hexanedione in rats: early morphological and functional changes in nerve fibers and neuromuscular junctions, *Neurotoxicology,* 2, 25, 1980.

27. **Chang, C. C., Chen, T. F., and Chuang, S-T.,** Influence of chronic neostigmine treatment on the number of acetylcholine receptors and the release of acetylcholine from the rat diaphragm, *J. Physiol.,* 230, 613, 1973.

28. **Cooper, G. P. and Manalis, R. S.,** Influence of heavy metals on synaptic transmission: a review, *Neurotoxicology,* 4, 69, 1983.

29. **Cooper, G. P. and Manalis, R. S.,** Interactions of lead and cadmium on acetylcholine release at the frog neuromuscular junction, *Toxicol. Appl. Pharmacol.,* 74, 411, 1984.

30. **Cooper, G. P. and Manalis, R. S.,** Heavy metals: effects on synaptic transmission, *Neurotoxicology,* 5, 247, 1984.

31. **Cooper, G. P., Suszkiw, J. B., and Manalis, R. S.,** Presynaptic effects of heavy metals, in *Cellular and Molecular Neutoroxicology,* Narahashi, T., Ed., Raven Press, New York, 1984, 1.

32. **DiVincenzo, G., Kaplan, C. J., and Dedinas, J.,** Characterization of the metabolites of methyl-*n*-butyl ketone, methyl isobutyl ketone and methyl ethyl ketone in guinea pig serum and their clearance, *Toxicol. Appl. Pharmacol.,* 36, 511, 1976.

33. **Dodge, F. A., Jr. and Rahamimoff, R.,** Cooperative action of Ca ions in transmitter release at the neuromuscular junction, *J. Physiol. (London),* 193, 419, 1967.

33a. **Dreisbach,** *Handbook of Poisoning: Prevention, Diagnosis and Treatment,* Lange Medical Publications, Los Altos, 1983.

34. **Duncan, C. J.,** Parallels between spontaneous release of transmitter at the neuromuscular junction and subcellular damage of muscle. Evidence for the underlying common involvement of intracellular Ca^{++}?, *Comp. Biochem. Physiol.,* 73A, 147, 1982.

35. **Eccles, J. C., Katz, B., and Kuffler, S. W.,** Effects of eserine on neuromuscular transmission, *J. Neurophysiol.,* 5, 211, 1942.

36. **Eccles, J. C. and MacFarlane, W. V.,** Actions of anticholinesterases on endplate potential of frog muscle, *J. Neurophysiol.,* 12, 59, 1949.

37. **Erulkar, S. D.,** The modulation of neurotransmitter release at synaptic junctions, *Rev. Physiol. Biochem. Pharmacol.,* 98, 63, 1983.

38. **Evans, M. H.,** Endplate potentials in frog muscle exposed to a synthetic pyrethroid, *Pest. Biochem. Physiol.,* 6, 547, 1976.

39. **Farley, J. M., Narahashi, T., and Holan, G.,** The mechanism of action of a DDT analog on the crayfish neuromuscular junction, *Neurotoxicology,* 1, 191, 1979.

40. **Fiskum, G. and Lehninger, A. L.,** The mechanisms and regulation of mitochondrial Ca^{++} transport, *Fed. Proc.,* 39, 2432, 1980.

41. **Fox, D. A., Lowndes, H. E., and Bierkamper, G. G.,** Electrophysiological techniques in neurotoxicology, in *Nervous System Toxicology,* Mitchell, C. L., Ed., Raven Press, New York, 1982, 299.

42. **Gage, P. W.,** The effect of methyl, ethyl and *n*-propyl alcohol on neuromuscular transmission in the rat, *J. Pharmacol. Exp. Ther.*, 150, 236, 1965.

43. **Gage, P. W., McBurney, R. N., and Schneider, G. T.,** Effects of some aliphatic alcohols on the conductance change caused by a quantum of acetylcholine at the toad end-plate, *J. Physiol.*, 244, 409, 1975.

44. **Ginsborg, B. L. and Jenkinson, D. H.,** Transmission of impulses to nerve and muscle, in *Neuromuscular Junction*, Zaimis, E., Ed., *Handbook of Experimental Pharmacology*, Vol. 42, Springer-Verlag, New York, 1976, 229.

45. **Glickman, A. H. and Casida, J. E.,** Species and structural variations affecting pyrethroid neurotoxicity, *Neurobehav. Toxicol. Teratol.*, 4, 793, 1982.

46. **Hobbiger, F.,** Pharmacology of anticholinesterase drugs, in *Neuromuscular Junction*, Zaimis, E., Ed., *Handbook of Experimental Pharmacology*, Vol. 42, Springer-Verlag, New York, 1976, 587.

47. **Hubbard, J. I. and Løyining, Y.,** The effects of hypoxia on neuromuscular transmission in a mammalian preparation, *J. Physiol.*, 185, 205, 1966.

48. **Johnson, M. K.,** The delayed neuropathy caused by some organophosphorus esters: mechanism and challenge, *CRC Crit. Rev. Toxicol.*, 3, 289, 1975.

49. **Johnson, M. K.,** Initiation of organophosphate-induced delayed neuropathy, *Neurobehav. Toxicol. Teratol.*, 4, 759, 1982.

50. **Juang, M. S.,** An electrophysiological study of the action of methylmercuric chloride and mercuric chloride on the sciatic nerve-sartorius muscle preparation of the frog, *Toxicol. Appl. Pharmacol.*, 37, 339, 1976.

51. **Juang, M. S. and Yonemura, K.,** Increased spontaneous transmitter release from presynaptic nerve terminal by methylmercuric chloride, *Nature (London)*, 256, 211, 1975.

52. **Katz, B.,** The Croonian lecutre: the transmission of impulse from nerve to muscle and the subcellular unit of synaptic activity, *Proc. R. Soc. London*, 155, 455, 1962.

53. **Katz, B.,** The release of neural transmitter substances, in *The Sherrington Lectures*, Vol. 10, Liverpool University Press, Liverpool, 1969.

54. **Katz, B. and Miledi, R.,** The nature of the prolonged endplate depolarization in anti-esterase treated muscle, *Proc. R. Soc. London B*, 192, 27, 1975.

55. **Katz, B. and Thesleff, S.,** On the factors which determine the amplitude of the "miniature end-plate potentials", *J. Physiol. (London)*, 137, 267, 1957.

56. **Khairy, M.,** Effects of chronic dieldrin ingestion on the muscular efficiency of rats, *Br. J. Ind. Med.*, 17, 146, 1960.

57. **Kober, T. E. and Cooper, G. P.,** Lead competitively inhibits calcium-dependent synaptic transmission in the bullfrog sympathetic ganglion, *Nature (London)*, 262, 704, 1976.

58. **Kolton, L. and Yaari, Y.,** Sites of action of lead on spontaneous release from motor nerve terminals, *Isr. J. Med. Sci.*, 18, 165, 1982.

59. **Kordas, M.,** An attempt at an analysis of the factors determining the time course of the endplate current. I. The effects of prostigmine and of the ratio Mg^{++} to Ca^{++}, *J. Physiol.*, 224, 317, 1972.

60. **Kordas, M.,** On the role of junctional cholinesterase in determining the time course of the end-plate current, *J. Physiol.*, 270, 133, 1977.

61. **Kostial, K. and Vouk, V. B.,** Lead ions and synaptic transmission in the superior cervical ganglion of the cat, *Br. J. Pharmacol.*, 12, 219, 1957.

62. **Kraatz, H. G. and Trautwein, W.,** Die wirkung von 2,4-dinitrophenol (DNP) auf die neuromuskuare erregungsubertragung, *Arch. Exp. Path. Pharmak.*, 231, 419, 1957.

63. **Kuba, K., Albuquerque, E. X., and Barnard, E. A.,** Diisopropylfluorophosphate: suppression of ionic conductance of the cholinergic receptor, *Science*, 181, 853, 1973.

64. **Kuba, K., Albuquerque, E. X., Daly, J., and Barnard, E. A.,** A study of the irreversible cholinesterase inhibitor, diisopropylfluorophosphate, on the time course of the end-plate currents in frog sartorius muscle, *J. Pharmacol. Exp. Ther.*, 189, 499, 1974.

65. **Laskowski, M. B. and Dettbarn, W.-D.,** An electrophysiological analysis of the effects of paraoxon at the neuromuscular junction, *J. Pharmacol. Exp. Ther.*, 210, 269, 1979.

66. **Laskowski, M. B. and Dettbarn, W.-D.,** Presynaptic effects of neuromuscular cholinesterase inhibition, *J. Pharmacol. Exp. Ther.*, 194, 351, 1975.

67. **Laskowski, M. B., Olson, W. H., and Dettbarn, W.-D.,** Initial ultrastructural abnormalities at the motor end plate produced by a cholinesterase inhibitor, *Exp. Neurol.*, 57, 13, 1977.

68. **Laskowski, M. B., Olson, W. H., and Dettbarn, W.-D.,** Ultrastructural changes at the motor end-plate produced by an irreversible cholinesterase inhibitor, *Exp. Neurol.*, 47, 290, 1975.

69. **Leonard, J. P. and Salpeter, M. M.,** Agonist-induced myopathy at the neuromuscular junction is mediated by calcium, *J. Cell Biol.*, 82, 811, 1979.

69a. **Lievremont, M., Barnier, J. V., and Potus, J.,** Gamma-hexachlorocyclohexane inhibition of the calcium-fluxes at the desensitized mouse neuromuscular junction, *Toxicol. Appl. Pharmacol.*, 76, 280, 1984.

69b. **Main,** personal observation, 1976.

70. **Manalis, R. S. and Cooper, G. P.,** Presynaptic and postsynaptic effects of lead at the frog neuromuscular junction, *Nature (London),* 243, 354, 1973.

71. **Manalis, R. S. and Cooper, G. P.,** Evoked transmitter release increased by inorganic mercury at frog neuromuscular junction, *Nature (London),* 257, 690, 1975.

72. **Manalis, R. S., Cooper, G. P., and Pomeroy, S. L.,** Effects of lead on neuromuscular transmission in the frog, *Brain Res.,* 294, 95, 1984.

73. **Marchi, M., Paudice, P., and Raiteri, M.,** Autoregulation of acetylcholine release in isolated hippocampal nerve endings, *Eur. J. Pharmacol.,* 73, 75, 1981.

74. **McLachlan, E. M.,** The statistics of transmitter release at chemical synapses, *Int. Rev. Physiol.,* 17, 49, 1978.

75. **Millington, W. R. and Bierkamper, G. G.,** Chronic triethyltin exposure reduces the resting membrane potential of rat soleus muscle, *Neurobehav. Toxicol. Teratol.,* 4, 255, 1982.

76. **Miyamoto, M. D.,** Hg^{++} causes neurotoxicity at an intracellular site following entry through Na and Ca channels, *Brain Res.,* 267, 375, 1983.

77. **Moore, K. E. and Brody, T. M.,** The effect of triethyltin on oxidative phosphorylation and mitochodrial adenosine triphosphate activation, *Biochem. Pharmacol.,* 6, 125, 1961.

78. **Moore, K. E. and Brody, T. M.,** The effect of triethyltin on mitochondrial swelling, *Biochem. Pharmacol.,* 6, 134, 1961.

79. **Murphy, S. D.,** Pesticides, in *Casarett and Doull's Toxicology,* 2nd ed., Doull, J., Klaassen, C. D., and Amdur, M. O., Eds., Macmillan, New York, 1980, 379.

80. **Murphy, S. D., Costa, L. G., and Wang, C.,** Organophosphate insecticide interactions at primary and secondary receptors, in *Cellular and Molecular Neurotoxicology,* Narahashi, T., Ed., Raven Press, New York, 1984, 165.

81. **Nachtman, J. P. and Couri, C.,** Biophysical and electrophysiological studies of hexanedione neurotoxicity, *Neurotoxicology,* 2, 541, 1981.

82. **Narahashi, T. and Haas, H. G.,** DDT: interaction with nerve membrane conductance changes, *Science,* 157, 1438, 1967.

83. **Narahashi, T.,** Effects of insecticides on excitable tissues, in *Advances in Insect Physiology,* Beament, J. W. L., Treherne, J. E., and Wigglesworth, V. B., Eds., Academic Press, New York, 1971, 1.

84. **Narahashi, T.,** Chemicals as tools in the study of excitable membranes, *Physiol. Rev.,* 54, 813, 1974.

85. **Narashashi, T.,** Nerve membrane sodium channels as the target of pyrethroids, in *Cellular and Molecular Neurotoxicology,* Narahashi, T., Ed., Raven Press, New York, 1984, 85.

86. **Porter, W. R., Dickins, J., Atchison, W. D., and Peterson, R. E.,** Effects of dose and dosing regimen on tissue distribution and elimination kinetics of [^{14}C] dithiobiuret in rats, *Neurotoxicology,* 4, 57, 1983.

87. **Publicover, S. J. and Duncan, C. J.,** The action of lindane in accelerating the spontaneous release of transmitter at the frog neuromuscular junction, *Naunyn-Schmiedeberg's Arch. Pharmacol.,* 308, 179, 1979.

88. **Publicover, S. J. and Duncan, C. J.,** The action of verapamil on the rate of spontaneous release of transmitter at the frog neuromuscular junction, *Eur. J. Pharmacol.,* PB54PB, 119, 1979.

89. **Publicover, S. J., Duncan, C. J., and Smith, J. L.,** The action of lindane in causing ultrastructural damage in frog skeletal muscle, *Comp. Biochem. Physiol.,* 1979.

90. **Rahamimoff, R.,** The regulation of intracellular calcium concentration and transmitter release, *Neurosci. Res. Prog. Bull.,* 15, 575, 1979.

91. **Redfern, P. and Thesleff, A.,** Action potential generation in denervated rat skeletal muscle. II. the action of tetrodotoxin, *Acta Physiol. Scand.,* 82, 70, 1971.

91a. **Reed, T. E.,** Acute effects of ethanol *in vivo* on neuromuscular transmission, *Pharmacol. Biochem. Behavior,* 13, 811, 1984.

92. **Richman, E. A. and Bierkamper, G. G.,** Histopathology of spinal cord, peripheral nerve, and soleus muscle of rats treated with triethyltin bromide, *Exp. Neurol.,* 86, 122, 1984.

93. **Sabri, M. I., Ederle, K., Holdsworth, C. H., and Spencer, P. S.,** Studies on the biochemical basis of distal axonopathies. II. Inhibition of fructose-6-phosphate kinase by neurotoxic hexacarbon compounds, *Neurotoxicology,* 1, 285, 1979.

94. **Salpeter, M. M., Kasprzak, H., Feng, H., and Fertuck, H.,** Endplates after esterase inactivation *in vivo:* correlation between esterase concentration, functional response and fine structure, *J. Neurocytol.,* 8, 95, 1979.

95. **Salpeter, M. M., Leonard, J. P., and Krasprzak, H.,** Agonist-induced postsynaptic myopathy, *Neurosci. Comment.,* 1, 77, 1982.

96. **Selwyn, M. J., Dawson, A. P., Stockdale, M., and Gains, N.,** Chloride-hydroxide exchange across mitochondrial, erthrocyte and artificial lipid membranes mediated by trialkyl- and triphenyltin compounds, *Eur. J. Biochem.,* 14, 120, 1970.

97. **Shankland, D. L.,** Neurotoxic action of chlorinated hydrocarbon insecticides, *Neurobehav. Toxicol. Teratol.,* 4, 805, 1982.

98. **Souyri, F. and Hoellinger, H.,** Neurotoxicity of pyrethrins in warm-blooded animals, *Toxicol. Eur. Res.,* 5, 103, 1983.

99. **Spencer, P. S. and Schaumberg, H. H.,** Experimental neuropathy produced by 2,5-hexanedione a major metabolite of the neurotoxic industrial solvent, methyl-*n*-butyl ketone, *J. Neurol. Neurosurg. Psychiatr.,* 38, 771, 1975.

100. **Spencer, P. S., Couri, D., and Schaumburg, H.H.,** *n*-Hexane and methyl *n*-butyl ketone, in *Experimental and Clinical Neurotoxicology,* Spencer, P. S. and Schaumburg, H. H., Eds., Williams & Wilkins, Baltimore, 1980, 456.

100a. **Spivak, C. E. and Albuquerque, E. X.,** Dynamic properties of the nicotinic acetylcholine receptor ionic channel complex: activation and blockade, in *Progress in Cholinergic Biology: Model Cholinergic Synapses,* Hanin, I. and Goldberg, A. M., Raven Press, New York, 1982, 323.

101. **Stanley, E. F. and Drachman, D. B.,** Denervation and the time course of resting membrane potential changes in skeletal muscle in vivo, *Exp. Neurol.,* 69, 253, 1980.

102. **Steinacker, A. and Zuazaga, D. C.,** Changes in neuromuscular junction endplate current time constants produced by sulfhydryl reagents, *Proc. Natl. Acad. Sci. U.S.A.,* 78, 7806, 1981.

103. **Stockdale, M., Dawson, A. P., and Selwyn, M. J.,** Effects of trialkyltin and triphenyltin compounds on mitochondrial respiration, *Eur. J. Biochem.,* 15, 342, 1970.

104. **Takeno, K., Nishimure, K., Parmentier, J., and Narahashi, T.,** Insecticide screening with isolated nerve preparations for structure-activity relationships, *Pest. Biochem. Physiol.,* 7, 486, 1977.

105. **Tan, L. P. and Ng, M. L.,** The toxic effects of trialkyltin compounds on nerve and muscle, *J. Neurochem.,* 29, 689, 1977.

106. **Tiedt, T. N., Albuquerque, E. X., Hudson, C. S., and Rash, J. E.,** Neostigmine-induced alterations at the mammalian neuromuscular junction. I. muscle contraction and electrophysiology, *J. Pharmacol. Exp. Ther.,* 205, 326, 1978.

107. **Tosteson, M. T. and Wieth, J. O.,** Tributyltin-mediated exchange diffusion of halides in lipid bilayers, *J. Gen. Physiol.,* 73, 789, 1979.

108. **van den Bercken, J.,** The action of allethrin on the peripheral nervous system of the frog, *Pest. Sci.,* 8, 692, 1977.

109. **van den Bercken, J., Akkermans, L. M. A., and van der Zalm, J. M.,** DDT-like action of allethrin in the sensory nervous system of *Xenopus** laevis, Eur. J. Pharmacol.,* 21, 95, 1973.

110. **van den Bercken, J., Kroese, A. B. A., and Akkermans, L. M. A.,** Effects of insecticides on the sensory nervous system, in *Neurotoxicology of Insecticides and Pheromones,* Narahashi, T., Ed., Plenum Press, New York, 1979, 183.

111. **Wachtel, R. E.,** Aliphatic alcohols increase the decay rate of glutamate-activated currents at the crayfish neuromuscular junction, *Br. J. Pharmacol.,* 83, 393, 1984.

112. **Wang, C. M., Narahashi, T., and Yamada, M.,** The neutotoxic action of dieldrin and its derivatives in the cockroach, *Pest. Biochem. Physiol.,* 1, 84, 1971.

113. **Wecker, L., Kiauta, T., and Dettbarn, W.-D.,** Relationship between acetylcholinesterase inhibition and the development of a myopathy, *J. Pharmacol. Exp. Ther.,* 206, 97, 1978.

114. **Wecker, L., Laskowski, M. B., and Dettbarn, W.-D.,** Neuromuscular dysfunction induced by acetyl-cholinesterase inhibition, *Fed. Proc.,* 37, 2818, 1978.

115. **Wieth, J. O. and Tosteson, M. T.,** Organotin-mediated diffusion of anions in human red cells, *J. Physiol.,* 73, 765, 1979.

116. **Williams, K. D., LoPachin, R. M., Atchison, W. D., and Peterson, R. E.,** Antagonism of dithiobiuret toxicity in rats, *Neurotoxicology,* 1985, in press.

117. **Wilson, D. F.,** Influence of presynaptic receptors on neuromuscular transmission in rat, *Am. J. Physiol.,* 242, 366, 1982.

118. **Winlow, W. and Usherwood, P. R. N.,** Electrophysiological studies of normal and degenerating mouse neuromuscular junctions, *Brain Res.,* 110, 447, 1976.

119. **Wouters, W., va den Bercken, J. and van Ginneken, A.,** Presynaptic action of the pyrethroid insecticide allethrin in the frog motor end plate, *Eur. J. Pharmacol.,* 43, 163, 1977.

120. **Wouters, W. and van den Bercken, J.,** Action of pyrethroids, *Gen. Pharmacol.,* 9, 387, 1978.

121. **Bierkamper, G. G.,** et al., unpublished.

122. **Blake, G., Dretchen, K., Valdes, J., and Bierkamper, G. G.,** unpublished.

123. **Atchison, W. D.,** personal communication,

INDEX

A

Acetylcholinesterase (AchE), 117, 128

Achlorophene, 60

Acrylamide, 60, 64, 77, 79
central-peripheral axonopathy caused by, 25—26
effects on spinal cord reflexes of, 39, 40

Acrylamide neuropathy, 45—47

Acrylamide neurotoxicity, 95—96

A/D conversion rate, 28

Age
development of SEPs and, 13—14
NI duration and latency and, 16
onset latency of NI peak in humans and, 15

Aldrin-transdiol (ATD), 113—115

Aliphatic alcohols, 122—125

Allethrin, 111, 112

Alpha-motoneurons, 36, 37

Alzheimer's disease, 21

Amplitude, and magnitude of sensation, 18

Amyotrophic lateral sclerosis, 21

Anesthesia, 6, 21

Anticholinesterase (ACh)
iontophoretic application of, 101, 114
in postsynaptic toxicity, 128

Anticholinesterase agents, synaptic toxicology of, 116—121

Antidromic activity, 120, 121

Arsenic trioxide, 62

B

Baboons
exposed to hexanedione, 25
first poststimulus sign of cortical activity in, 13

Bandpass, 28

Barbiturate anesthesia, 6

Bicuculline, 22

Bioenergetic pathways, in postsynaptic toxicity, 128

Body size
NI duration and latency and, 16
onset latency of NI peak in humans and, 15

Body temperature, influence of anesthetics on, 22

Brain function, and somatic sensation, 16

Brainstem auditory evoked response (BAER), 9

"Branch point failure", of nerve conduction, 52

Bregma, 14

Broadmann's area, cross species comparisons for, 10

Brown-Schuster myograph, 81

Buffering processes, in synaptic toxicity, 127

C

Calcium, 101, 103

Calcium channels, in synaptic toxicity, 127

Carbon disulfide, 64

Carpal tunnel syndrome, waveform morphology of, 18

Cationic interactions, 106

Cats
kindling of cortex in, 20
median nerve stimulation of, 10
peak latency of SEP components in, 11
poststimulus sign of cortical activity in, 14
SEPs recorded from, 19
thalamocortical afferents in, 9

"Central conduction time", 9, 22, 28

Central nervous system (CNS), axon-myelin relationship in, 53

Cholinergic receptor density, 120

Clioquinol, 25, 60, 64

"Closed field" geometry, 9

Cockroach, synaptic transmission in CNS of, 113

Coma, SEP waves in, 21

Compound action potential (CAP) response, 47

Conduction block, 57—59

Conduction velocity
axon-myelin relationship in, 53
conditions and agents producing changes in, 58
determination of, 82
effect of neurotoxic agents on, 56
conduction block, 57—59
decreased conduction velocity, 59
increased excitability, 59
remyelination, 59—60
geometry of, 52—53
history of, 52, 53
measurement of
clinical, 54—55
experimental, 55—56
as measure of neurotoxicity, 65
neurotoxic studies, 61—64
role of myelin in, 54

Cortex
SEPs produced in, 5, 7
somatosensory map of, 14

Cortical myoclonus, 20

Cutaneous receptors
effect of chemical toxins on, 79—80
effect of neurotoxic drugs on, 80
mechanoreceptors, 74—76
nociceptors, 76
recording setup for study of, 81
thermoreceptors, 76

Cyclohexane, 25

D

DDT, synaptic toxicology of, 116—117

Demonstration-type studies, 27

Demyelinating disease, 18

Demyelination, and remyelination, 59

DFF, 64, 118
Diagnostic aids, SEPs as, 21
Dieldrin, 113
Diesel exhaust, neonatal exposure to, 23
Diisopropylfluorophosphate (DFP) mononeuropathy,
    93—95
Diphenyl, 64
Dithiobiuret (DTG), 121—122
Dorsal column system, 3
Dorsal root ganglia, 72, 73
Dorsal root potential (DRP), 38
    effect of ethanol on, 41
    electrode placement for recording of, 43
Dorsal root reflex (DRR)
    defined, 38
    electrode placement for recording of, 43
Dorsal root responses, 38, 47—48
Down's Syndrome, 20
Drugs, facilitatory, 88
"Dying-back" process, 93

E

EDO, 116
Endplate potential (EPP), depressed by lead, 101
Epilepsy, 20
Ethanol, 64, 78
    effects on neurotransmission at rat neuromuscular
        junction, 122
    effect on spinal cord reflexes, 41
    prolongation of MEPCs caused by, 124
Ethyl acetate, 25
Evoked potentials, visual, 16
Excitatory postsynaptic potential (EPSP), 7, 38

F

Facilitatory drugs, 88
Far-field SEPs (FFSEPs), 8—9, 13
    cross-species comparisons, 10
    in neurotoxicity studies, 26
Fast fibers, 2
Fentanyl, 22
Frog nerve muscle, 52, 53
Frog neuromuscular junction, 104

G

GABA
    PAD mediated by, 38
    SEPs stimulated by, 22
Gender differences, in SEPs, 16—17
Generators, and first positive peak of cortical origin
    in humans, 15—16
Glucocorticoids, to delay neuropathy development,
    95
Golgi tendon organs, 74
Gyri

potentials distorted by, 12
in surface topography of recorded potentials, 10

H

Haarscheibs, 74, 75
Halogenated hydrocarbons, 113—115
Hexacarbon neurotoxicity, 60
Hexacarbons, neuropathy produced by, 24—25
Hexachlorophene, 63
n-Hexane, 63
Hexanedione, 125—126
Homosynaptic depression, 45, 46
Hormonal processes, and development of SEPs, 23
H-reflex
    clinical study of, 39
    effect of ethanol on, 41
Humans
    median nerve stimulation of, 10
    peak latency of SEP components in, 11
    poststimulus sign of cortical activity in, 14
    thalamocortical afferents in, 9
Huntington's disease, 20

I

Iminodipropionitrile (IDPN), 96
    effect on spinal cord reflexes of, 39
    microtubule-neurofilament interactions altered by,
        60
Insecticides, synaptic toxicology of
    anticholinesterase agents, 117—121
    DDT, 116—117
    halogenated hydrocarbons, 113—115
    lindane, 115—116
    pyrethroids, 111—113
Intracranial recordings, 9
IPSPs, 7
Isoniazid, 64
Isopotential maps, 5, 6

J

Joint receptors, 76

K

Kitten, see also Cats, 13
Krause's end-bulbs, 76

L

Lanthanum, 109
Latency coefficients, for median nerve SEPs, 4
Lead, 61—62
    competitive interaction with calcium, 101

synaptic toxicology of, 101—105
Lead toxicity, 23
Lindane, 115—116
Linear variable differential transformer (LVDT), 84
Lissencephalic brains, 10, 12
Lysophosphatidyl choline, 56, 60, 64

M

Macaque median nerve, 5, 6
Malnutrition, and development of SEPs, 23
Mauthner axons, 58
Mechanoreceptors
  cutaneous, 74—76
  isolation and recording of, 82—84
  of skeletal muscle, 74
Median nerve
  human, 9
  macaque, 5, 6
  SEPs following electrical stimulation of, 5, 6
  SEPs recorded following electrical stimulation of, 17
  stimulation of, 9
Median nerve SEPs, latency coefficients for, 4
Medulla, in somatosensory pathways, 2
Meissner's corpuscles, 76
Membrane, in postsynaptic toxicity, 128
Membrane fluidity, 125
Mercury, 61
  effect of channel blocking agents on, 107
  synaptic toxicology of, 105—109
Methyl alcohol, 123
Methyl-ethyl ketone, 25
Methyl mercury, 60, 61
  effect on MEPPs, 109
  MEPP frequency enhanced by, 106
  presynaptic effects of, 108
Methylprednisolone, 95
Miniature end-plate potentials (MEPPs)
  effects of lanthanum on, 109
  effects of methylmercury on, 109
  increased by cadmium, 104
  increased by lead, 101
Monkeys
  exposed to acrylamide, 26
  median nerve stimulation of, 10
  peak latency of SEP components in, 11
  poststimulus sign of cortical activity in, 14
  thalamocortical afferents in, 9
Monosynaptic reflex (MSR), 36, 37
  effect of acrylamides on, 39
  effect of ethanol on, 41
  electrode placement for recording of, 43
  testing protocols, 36
    inhibition, 46—47
    unconditioned response, 44
Motor nerve endings
  neurotoxicology of, 93
  post-drug repetition in, 88, 89
  post-tetanic repetition in, 88, 90

recording procedures for, 93
repetitive discharges of
  conditioned by edrophonium, 91
  conditioned by high frequency stimulation, 92
responsiveness model for, 89
  anesthesia, 90
  surgical preparation, 90—92
Multiple sclerosis (MS), 21, 58
Muscle spindles
  measurement of position for, 82
  role of, 72—74
  sensory nerve terminal function determined by, 80
Myelin, 54
Myelin sheath, 52

N

Neostigmine methylsulfate, 118
Neurohumoral transmission, toxicology of, 100
Neurological disorders, SEP changes in, 18
Neuropsychological deficit, prediction of, 21
Neurosurgery, 19
Neurotoxicity, delayed, 40
Neurotoxicology, see also Synaptic toxicology
  SEPs in, 22—27
  tests of nerve responsiveness in
    acrylamide neurotoxicity, 95—96
    iminodipropionitrile, 96
    organophosphate neuropathy, 93—95
    systemic organophosphate neuropathy, 95
    vincristine, 96
Neurotransmitters, in postsynaptic toxicity, 128
Nitrous oxide, 22
Nociceptors, 76
NRDC 119, 112

O

2-Octanol, 63
Onset latencies, 28
Organophosphate neuropathy, 93—95
Organophosphorous (OP) agents, 39, 77
Organotin compounds, 110

P

Pacinian corpuscles, 79
Pain, inability to experience, 17
Paraoxon, 119
Paraoxon myopathy, 120
Parietal lesions, and SEPs, 20
Peak latencies, 28
Peak to peak amplitudes, 28
Pentobarbital, 22
Perception, relationship of SEPs to, 17—18
Peripheral nerve, electrical stimulation of, 2—3
Peroneal nerve, stimulation of, 7, 18

Pharmacology, of SEPs, 21—22
Phenol, 58
Phenylmercuric acetate, 60
Picrotoxin, 22
Polychlorinated biphenyls, 64
Polysynaptic reflexes (PSR), 36, 37
Postjunctional receptors, 128
Postsynaptic inhibition, 36, 37, 46
Postsynaptic targets, 100
Post-tetanic potentiation (PTP), 36, 37
  effect of acrylamides on, 39
  tests of, 44
Potentials, measurement of, 44
Presynaptic inhibition, 36—38, 46
Presynaptic targets, 100
Primary afferent depolarization (PAD), 36
  antidromic potentials and, 38
  effect of ethanol on, 41
Primary afferent terminals (PATs), 39
Primary sensory neuron, 72
Proprioceptive sensation, 17
Proprioceptor function, 77—79
n-Propyl alcohol, 123
Pyrethroid insecticides, 111—113
Pyridine-2-aldoxime methiodide (2-PAM), 119, 120

Q

Quipazine, 40, 46

R

Rabbit, 13
Raccoons, 10—11
Rats
  exposed to acrylamide, 26
  map of somatosensory cortex in, 14
  median nerve stimulation of, 10
  peak latency of SEP components in, 11
  primary somatosensory cortex of, 13
  somatosensory system of, 12
  thalamocortical afferents in, 9
Recording configurations, for rat SEPs, 14, 15
Recurrent inhibition, 36, 37, 46
Reference electrode, "indifferent", 9
Reflexes, see Spinal cord reflexes
Remyelination, 59—60
Reye's syndrome, 21
Rodents, see Rats
Ruffini endings, 73, 75

S

SAI receptors, 74, 75, 79, 80
Sarin, 39
Schwann cells, 53
Sciatic nerve, stimulation of, 7
Screening, 5, 23

Senile dementia, 21
Sensory afferents, 72
Sensory nerve terminal function, 80—84
Sensory receptors
  cutaneous, 74—76
  joint, 76
  muscle, 72—74
  toxicology of, 76
    cutaneous receptor function, 79—80
    proprioceptor function, 77—79
  visceral, 76
Sheep, 13
Slow fibers, 2
Sodium channels, after demyelination, 57
Soleus muscle proprioceptors, recording setup for
    study of, 83
Soman, 39, 80
Somatosensory cortex, cutaneous representation in,
    13
Somatosensory dysfunction, 5
Somatosensory evoked potentials (SEPs)
  abnormalities of, 19
  exposed to clioquinol, 64
  interpretation of
    changes in neurological disorders, 18—20
    relationship to perception, 17—18
  major peaks of, 4
  phenomenology of, 3
    development of, 13—16
    far-field potentials, 8—9
    gender differences in, 16—17
    peak nomenclature, 4—8
    species comparison, 10—13
  recorded from cats, 19
  relative latencies for, 11
  use of, 2
    diagnostic, 21
    in neurotoxicology, 22—27
    pharmacological, 21—22
    surgical monitoring, 21
Somatosensory evoked potentials (SEPs) studies,
    27—28
Somatosensory pathways, 2, 3
Spatiotemporal properties, of SEPs, 5
Spectral analysis, 28
Spinal cord reflexes
  dorsal root response, 36, 38
  toxicology of
    chemical agents, 38—41
    drugs, 41
  toxicology studies
    dorsal root response, 47—48
    general in vitro procedures, 42
    general in vivo procedures, 41—42
    measurement of potentials, 44
    monosynaptic reflex testing protocols, 44—47
    stimulating and recording techniques, 42—43
  ventral root response, 36
Spinothalamic system, 3
Statistical analyses, 27
Steroids, 78, 79

Sulfhydryl binding, 106
Sural nerve, stimulation of, 7
Synaptic toxicology, 100
   of aliphatic alcohols, 122—125
   of dithiobiuret, 121
   of 2,5-hexanedione, 125—126
   of insecticides
      anticholinesterase agents, 117—121
      DDT, 116—117
      halogenated hydrocarbons, 113—115
      lindane, 115—116
      pyrethroids, 111—113
   mechanisms of, 127—128
   metals
      lead, 101—105
      mercury, 105—109
      organotin compounds, 110

T

Tabun, 39
Tactile stimulation, 17
Tail, stimulation of, 12
Temperature, inability to experience, 17
Tetradotoxin, 57—59
Thermoreceptors, 76
Threshold stimulation, 17
Tibial nerve, stimulation of, 7, 18, 20
TOCP, 39
Toluene, 63
Tooth pulp, electrical stimulation of, 8, 17
Toxicological studies, see also Synaptic toxicology,
   27
Toxic substances, perinatal exposure to, 23
Transmitter release, statistical parameters for, 102
Triamcinolone, 79, 95

Triethyltin (TET), 110
Trigeminal nerve, stimulation of, 7
Trimethyltin (TMT), 24
Tri-*ortho*-cresyl phosphate, 95
"t" tests, 27
Twitch response, 89

V

Variability analysis, 28
Velocity sensitivity, measurement of, 82
Ventral root responses
   monosynaptic reflex (MSR), 36, 37
   polysynaptic reflex (PSR), 36, 37
Vibrissae, 12
Vincristine, 64, 77—80, 96
Visceral receptors, 76
Visual system, and lead toxicity, 24

W

Waveform
   generators of, 5
   in phenomenology of SEPs, 3
   topographical distribution of, 28
Waveform morphologies, 7
   of carpal tunnel syndrome, 18
   produced by higher-intensity stimulation, 18, 19
"W" response, 25

Z

Zinc acetate, 62
Zinc pyridinethione, 60